RETHINKING HAND SAFETY

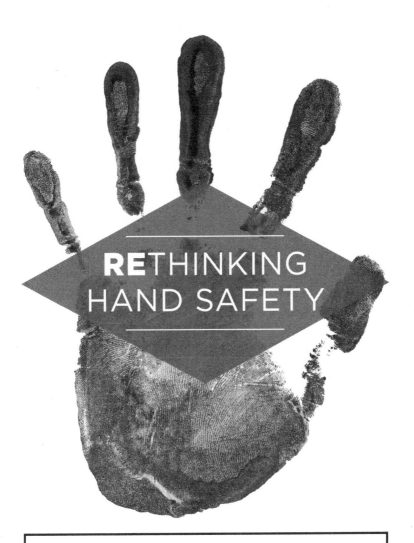

RETHINKING
HAND SAFETY

MYTHS, TRUTHS, AND PROVEN PRACTICES

JOE GENG

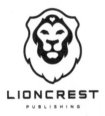

LIONCREST
PUBLISHING

RETHINKING HAND SAFETY
Myths, Truths, and Proven Practices

ISBN   978-1-5445-0625-8 *Paperback*
        978-1-5445-0626-5 *Ebook*

PRINTED IN CANADA

To my dad, Frank Geng, whose life's work and
passion was protecting workers' hands.

CONTENTS

ACKNOWLEDGMENTS

This book could not have been created without much research and input from people throughout the safety industry, and I have many to thank.

Let me start with the dedicated employees at Superior Glove, who have given me such support throughout this project and who work every day to make people safer.

I drew invaluable advice from specific interviews conducted with a large number of true experts. Let me thank them for their ready cooperation and wisdom: Marissa Afton, Syed Ahmed, Ken Ashfield, Louis Bevoc, Jennifer Boychuk, Jean Casey, Samuel Cunard, Ray Dibello, Dan Duffey, Derek Eversdyke, Chris Garrels, Maria Gonzalez, Matthew Hallowell, Jamie Hermann, Michael Johannesson, Thomas Krause, Danielle Kretschmer, Angela Lambert, Lorell Leitze, Timothy Ludwig, Simon MacInnis, Dennis Mehas, John Morawetz, Mary Sue Mumma, Steve Patterson, Charles Piper, Justin Raymond, Steve Roberts, Justin Tripp, and Chris Urbach.

Let me give special thanks to my very dedicated and talented book team, which included editor, Marc Porter Zasada, and publishing manager, Ellie Cole. Untiring consultants Delaney King, Lori Fleming, and Nedra Weinreich put in many hours of solid thinking and research. Research assistance was also provided by the very able Kristen Lightner and Chandra Lye. John Galvin and Caroline Bermudez did a fabulous job conducting interviews.

Finally, let me thank my wonderful wife, Julie, children Sebastian, Xavier, and Alexander for their endless patience and faith in me and support for my work.

INTRODUCTION

THE THREE KINDS OF COMPANIES

Usually, it's obvious.

When I walk onto a shop floor, I almost always know if I'm visiting the best kind of company, the worst kind of company, or a company struggling to get things right.

In my world, only those three kinds of companies exist. It doesn't matter if they're doing auto assembly, running canning lines, making jet engine parts, refining oil, or cutting sheet metal.

I visit these companies because it's my job to help them decide what kind of work gloves to buy—a vital, often difficult decision that will directly affect the safety of everyone on the shop floor. A decision that can save fingers. Hands. Livelihoods. Even lives.

If I'm visiting the best kind of company, the shop's well-lit. You could eat your dinner off the floor. The equipment's spotless and clearly maintained. I feel a sense of order, and I see a labeled place for everything. Whiteboards with production goals hang next to bright, detailed safety signs in multiple languages. The PPE (personal protective equipment) is obviously fresh, up to date, and worn by everyone.

In the best kind of companies, the workers themselves look relaxed and generally happy. They come up to chat, eager to engage and answer my questions.

In the best kind of companies, the workers realize I'm there because management actually cares about their safety. That gives us an immediate bond. I can ask, "Is this glove working for you?" and I'll get a straight answer, like, "Hey, this glove has no grip, so I never use it, even though I know I'm supposed to."

Then we figure out a solution. Together.

LIKE WALKING INTO A DIVE BAR

The worst kind of company will try to prevent me from touring the shop floor at all. They don't want prying eyes. They don't want advice on the best glove for a particular job. They just want to talk price.

If I do manage to get down to the floor, I feel like an unwelcome stranger entering a dive bar. It's dimly lit. Tools are scattered. Metal shavings litter the floor. I'll see lubricating oil pooling under grimy machinery. Workers will avoid my eye, and I can see they're asking, "Is this some new management guy sent to give us trouble?"

These workers aren't just suspicious, they're visibly grim. Unhappy. Resigned.

If the workers in the worst kind of company even use their PPE, it's cheap, filthy, and out of date. Gloves are old and randomly chosen, with the same worn, greasy leather used for handing sharp metal, pouring corrosive chemicals, or running saws. The company probably has an official policy for wearing protection, but it's hardly enforced or encouraged—so I'll see people reluctantly pulling on their protection as I enter and radioing ahead to others. I can see them thinking, "Oh, it's some kind of BS safety inspection, so we'd better make a show of it."

At the worst kind of companies, safety signs are nonexistent or vague. They say things like "Use Caution!" but everywhere I look, I see little evidence of caution.

Everywhere I look at the worst companies, I see tragedy close at hand.

TRYING TO GET IT RIGHT

The third kind of company is harder to spot, but maybe it's the kind of company most likely to use this book.

That's the kind of company struggling to get it right. The kind of company that cares, but doesn't know how to move forward. That wants to develop a genuine culture of safety, but doesn't see how to make it happen.

I'm thinking of an automotive parts plant where a manager takes me down to the shop floor to show me workers cutting metal parts. They have gloves with good cut protection, but they're using a cutting fluid that penetrates the gloves over time. Because the gloves are clumsy, they often take them off to handle small parts—despite signs saying "Always wear your gloves." Long-term exposure to cutting fluids can cause serious health issues, and the manager's genuinely worried about his workers.

He says to me, "This has been going on for twenty years, but I don't know how to fix it."

I'm thinking of a construction company that sends out hundreds of workers to multiple building sites. Some workers get a safety talk before they start, and some don't. Some bring their own gloves, and some get cheap gloves issued to them on an "as needed" basis. Plenty think they're too tough or experienced to follow formal safety procedures. The newbies, wanting to fit in, usually follow their lead.

The company employs a full-time safety manager, but he says to me, "I really have no idea how to reach these guys."

At this third kind of company, you find good practices here and there, but not everywhere. You find supervisors who give a safety talk to their teams every morning and supervisors who have never given a safety talk in their lives. You find dangerous equipment tagged and locked out when not being used alongside dangerous equipment left unlocked and unattended while the operator grabs lunch. There's no overall program that drives safety all the way through the organization. There's no systematic hazard assessment. There's no measurement of results.

At the best kind of company, I'm there because management has asked, "How can we do this better?"

At the worst kind of company, I'm there because they asked, "How can we do this cheaper?"

At the third kind of company, management honestly wants to know, "How can we get some kind of control over this situation?"

I'm writing this book to make a difference at all three kinds of companies. *Because at all three, regardless of the attitudes of management, hands matter.* Because every day, every hour, someone trying to earn a living injures a hand—bones crushed, fingers lost, skin burned, or a whole hand dismembered in a way that *could have been prevented.*

HOW THIS BOOK CAME ABOUT

As of this writing, my family's company has been making work gloves for 109 years.[1] We sell to automakers like Honda, Toyota, and General Motors. We supply oil and gas companies like Shell Oil, Nabors Drilling, and Jacobs Engineering. We create gloves for huge construction companies like Bechtel, innovative aerospace companies like Bombardier and SpaceX, and major food processors like Tyson Foods.

All around the globe, our representatives, R&D teams, and hand-safety consultants spend their careers looking for ways to make hands safer. They attend conferences. Hunt down new materials. Dig into statistics. Walk every kind of shop floor. As a result, we make—no kidding—over 1,000 different kinds of gloves in over 5,000 SKUs.

This book arises out of the passion and experience of everyone on our team; the lessons we've learned from the best companies; the advice we've sought from acclaimed safety experts and behavioral psychologists; reviews of the best academic studies; interviews with our most knowledgeable clients; and extensive talks with workers, supervisors, and independent safety trainers.

In this book, we'll get way beyond "What gloves should I buy?" to "What causes someone to act safely or not act safely?" We'll discuss cognitive biases and illegitimate statistics. We'll talk about managing up and managing down. Infrastructure dos and don'ts. But overall this book will be driven by one simple question:

What actually works?

Not what *might* work. Not what *should* work. Not what people *think* works. But what strategies, policies, processes, attitudes, training, and decisions *actually work* to reduce or eliminate hand injuries to workers out there in the real world: The people feeding stampers. Running lathes. Holding jackhammers. Welding beams. Handling acids. Working pile drivers.

The people whose hands represent their livelihood. And build our world.

MIND-FOCUSING STATS

It may shock you to learn that in the United States, workplace injuries cost more than all cancers combined—an estimated $250 billion annually. The hand is the most commonly injured part of the upper body,[2] with about 170,000 reported industrial hand injuries a year.[3] Each injury costs companies around US $10,200 in worker's comp,[4] along with five days' lost work, OSHA reports, and so on. You do the math.[5]

Overall, OSHA estimates a four to six dollar return for every dollar invested in safety—when that investment is actually made.[6][7]

Those numbers, of course, represent only the costs to companies and insurance funds. They don't account for the people who can no longer work after losing a hand. Or who develop lifelong disabilities from absorbing chemicals into their skin, or who can't button up their own shirt after losing some fingers.

In 2015, at one of America's largest poultry processors, they reported seventeen hand amputations.[8] That's more than one a month. That's seventeen real people who were crippled for life, in one year alone. As in, *they lost a hand.*

WHO SHOULD READ THIS BOOK

Mostly this book is for safety managers—at companies of any size, from a small machine shop in a small town up to a GM plant in Michigan or an oil rig out in the North Sea.

It's for safety managers who don't want to read through a hundred academic studies, but still want to get to zero injuries—or who have already read a bunch of studies, but don't believe there *is* such a thing as zero injuries.

It's for safety managers who may have been trained for the job—or who may have been thrown into their role because no one else raised their hand at a meeting or seemed willing to develop a plan.

But truly, this book is for *any kind of manager who cares* and finds themselves responsible for workers in manufacturing, construction, mining, food processing, healthcare, oil and gas, road maintenance, utility maintenance, transportation, or any other dangerous environment.

It's for any manager who has seen previous safety initiatives fail.

Any manager who wants to see how others fixed their failures.

Any member of a safety committee who really wants to move the ball forward.

Any middle manager who wants to change the attitude of upper management.

Any CEO who wants to change the attitude of their board, their colleagues, their middle managers, *and* their work teams.

In fact, this book is for anyone who wants to stand up and say, "Hey, we don't have to take cuts, crushes, lacerations, and burns for granted. It's not 'just part of the job.' It's not 'just part of life in this company.' We don't have to accept any 'natural rate of injury.' People are being hurt who don't need to be hurt, because yes, something can be done. Plenty of companies have figured out how to reduce or eliminate these kinds of injuries. Let's see how they did it, then let's make this place better."

GETTING BEYOND FRUSTRATION

Of course, maybe you've made that speech in the past, and you think you tried your damnedest, and your hand injury rate still didn't go down. Or you couldn't get funding. Or no one seemed to listen. Maybe you're at the point where you're thinking, "I just can't help these guys."

Well, a major goal of this book is to get you past the natural frustration of being a safety manager. I want to do that by helping you understand the underlying psychology and culture of safety. That means I won't shy away from questions like:

"Why don't people follow the rules?"

"Why didn't he see the sign right next to the damn machine?"

"Why don't these guys put the guards down on the blade *before* they run lumber through it? Isn't that, like, obvious?"

"Why would anyone not wear gloves when they're handing sheet metal? Are they idiots?"

"How can I change people?"

"How can I change a whole company of people?"

"How can I get serious money for training?"

"How can I make the CEO care?"

That means diving into the psychology of both workers and managers. It means getting beyond "common sense" to see the cognitive blocks that prevent safety at all levels of an organization.

In fact, a whole chapter is devoted to the mysterious psychology of safety.

DOING IT RIGHT, AGAIN AND AGAIN

One theme that runs through this book ain't sexy, but it's fundamental. So I might as well get it right out on the table.

That theme is *consistency*.

As I talked to folks across industries, and even within industries, I discovered that safety practices were anything but consistent. At one metal-handling facility they do it this way. At the facility next door they do it that way. This machine has all kinds of safety guards, and the next machine's got bare flying gears. One supervisor makes everyone wear gloves and the other supervisor thinks gloves are annoying. Somebody orders great new gloves, and six months later somebody else goes back to ordering the old cheap, crappy kind.

Don't tell me that government regulations create consistency, because they can't and they don't. Government regulations are only table stakes; it's how you play the game that matters. Only the people onsite who care—and care for years and years—can create the standards and culture that lead to real safety.

CONSISTENT INCONSISTENCIES

Training is probably the least consistent factor of all.

One VP starts a big safety training initiative and the next VP drops it. Jim does the training this way and Jane does it that way. Carl has never done safety training, but he gets the assignment because he knows how to do the work. Unfortunately, Carl can't really understand why anyone would get hurt doing what he does, as long as they're not outright idiots. Pete is tasked with training, but Pete doesn't really believe that you can *train* people to be safe, at all: "Hey, if their mommas didn't teach them to be safe, there's nothing I can do for them now."

As a result, one new hire gets a whole lot of random Power-Point shows, and the next gets nothing but a good luck pat on the back.

There's a reason the training chapter takes up a good chunk of this book. Plenty of hand-safety training doesn't work. We'll dig into the reasons and the ways of doing it right.

The Wheels

Then there's the problem of reinventing the wheel.

Tragically, lessons learned within industries are often not passed around. As a result, even safety managers who become passionate about their jobs often must reinvent the wheel when it comes to training and organizational engagement—despite the tried-and-true blueprints out there, maybe at a competitor, or maybe at another plant owned by the same company, just waiting to be tapped.

The Fires

Then there's the problem of putting out fires instead of looking at the big picture.

Even safety managers who wake up at 3 a.m. worrying about the hands of their workers often find themselves focused only on the latest disaster—say, those dangerous gears that grabbed somebody's finger last week—without ever stepping back to look at all the *potential* hazards in the workplace, then developing a repeatable approach to solving them.

THE LONG-TERM STUFF

To get at these problems, this book will look at much more than the mechanics of hand safety. We'll look at how to create organization-wide hand-safety processes, organization-wide safety cultures, and how to involve actual workers in actual safety planning.

Sexy or not, we'll look at how to create *consistency*. That means chapters on hazard assessments, on keeping stats, and on creating a meaningful company culture around safety. All developed with experts who have been there.

In other words: not just easy short-term tactics, but hard, long-term strategies.

Proven strategies.

HOW THIS BOOK WILL CHANGE YOU

Ultimately, I want this book to change you. I want it to change the way you approach safety—especially hand safety, but all safety. I want it to give you confidence that you completely "get it" and then to *rethink* the whole topic at your company.

Toward that end, this book tries to offer you all the key tools in a small volume. It's intended to arm you with the critical data, the essential psychological facts, case studies, and proven methodologies to make a real difference in the lives of your workers.

When you're done working through this book, you should *immediately* see how to greatly improve hand safety in your workplace, regardless of your industry, and regardless of your previous knowledge.

You should then be capable of creating your own realistic, go-forward plan. A plan that avoids the common pitfalls of the numberless safety programs that cost time and money and energy but failed to make real progress. On this book's supporting website at www.rethinkinghandsafety.com, you will find a checklist which can help.

WHAT'S NOT IN THIS BOOK

That said, you're not holding an encyclopedia. Here's some stuff that's beyond our scope here:

- You will not find first-aid instructions, or specific post-injury reporting standards within these pages, as those topics are well covered elsewhere and may be highly specific to your industry.
- You will not find much discussion of government regulations or government reporting requirements—again, just table stakes, particular to your industry, and well covered elsewhere.

I talk a lot about how to train for hand safety, but I do not present an actual hand-safety training curriculum. Curricula should also be highly customized, but I'll point you to resources you can download.

In fact, on the website at www.rethinkinghandsafety.com, you will find lots of linked resources, including hazard assessment forms, curriculums, and glove-selection information.

TWO INSPIRATIONS

I also hope this book will inspire you.

If you have picked up this little tome and read this far, it means you have the chance to do a great deal of good in the world.

You have the chance to save the hand of a human being, along with their livelihood, and possibly their life.

Indeed, since you have the chance to prevent disasters *before* they occur, your opportunity for good is *greater* than that given to the most skilled surgeon or altruistic charity.

Throughout the book, I will be quoting two men who have inspired me over the years. The first is Paul O'Neill, former CEO of Alcoa, who completely revolutionized safety across his global organization—and made Alcoa far more successful at the same time.

On his very first investor call, O'Neill shocked the financial world and briefly tanked his stock by saying, "If you want to see how I'm doing, look at my safety record." Not his profitability, not his sales, but his safety record. "Don't budget safety," said O'Neill to his managers, "Just do it." At first they thought he was nuts. Then they saw he was right. I'll tell you the whole story later.

The second is David White, Senior VP of the global supply chain at Campbell's Soup for ten years, who reduced lost-time injuries by 90 percent and changed the way his entire industry thought about safety.

Whether you work at the best kind of company, the worst kind of company, or a company struggling to do better—let's learn from White and O'Neill and the many others who will lead our way.

Together, let's save some hands.

CHAPTER ONE

WHY BAD THINGS HAPPEN TO GOOD HANDS

Robotics engineers dream great dreams of duplicating the hand, but still can't design one that delicately picks a strawberry like the lowest-paid field worker.

No other part of the body has the hand's dexterity. Its sensitivity. Its muscle intelligence. We eat with our hands, dress with our hands, touch our lovers with our hands.

Built with no less than twenty-seven separate bones connected by a complex network of tendons, ligaments, and muscles, this perfectly evolved machine offers a range of motion utterly unique in its beauty and capability.

The human hand is not a minor miracle, it's a major miracle.

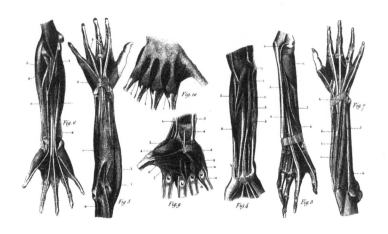

Strangely, however, hand injuries are often taken for granted. I see it all the time…

The boss of an oil rig in California says to one of my territory managers, "These are tough guys out here. They don't care if their hands get bruised, and we only break a few fingers a year. It's not a huge deal. We just fix them up and actually they go back out and start working again with their broken finger." It's clear that the rig boss keeps no records on mere hand injuries. Performs no follow-up to see if the worker lost range of motion, or the broken fingers mended crooked. For sure, he's not willing to upgrade to more expensive gloves. A week later, we learn that a worker on the same rig had a finger cut off while wearing fifty-cent nitrile gloves that offered no real protection.

We're visiting a sheet metal manufacturer where workers handle sharp edges all day long. In the shop, we see that the old guys aren't using any gloves at all. We actually see one worker in his mid-fifties get cut on a big piece of metal. When we ask why he's not wearing gloves, he replies, "I don't need that kind of stuff. When I get cut, I just use some crazy glue and gaffer tape." He holds up his hands, which are completely covered in scars, callouses, and some burns. Nearby there's a younger worker, and we can see him thinking, "If I ask for gloves, my boss will think I'm a sissy." '

IT SUCKS TO "JUST LOSE A FINGER OR TWO".

Anything as complex as the hand is also extremely difficult to repair. Even if you "just lose a finger or two." Never mind having your whole hand crushed.

Crazy glue and gaffer tape rarely solve the problem.

If a great violinist injures a hand, we all know it's a tragedy. But few people seem to realize how a hand injury can deeply impact *anyone's* life: prevent them from brushing their teeth, picking a flower, preparing food, handling a fishing pole, changing a baby.

In our training sessions we sometimes tape up one or two fingers on a worker's hand, as if the fingers had been lost—then ask the worker to button their shirt, sign their name, or tie their shoe.

Try it. Tape a couple fingers of your good hand together and try to sign a check, eat, or button your shirt. How about playing a guitar? Picking flowers? Holding your child?

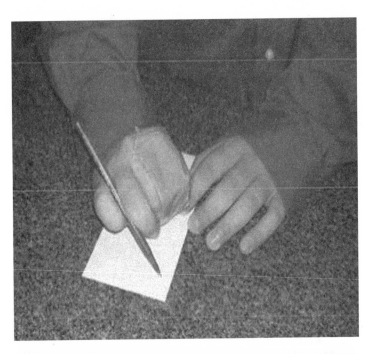

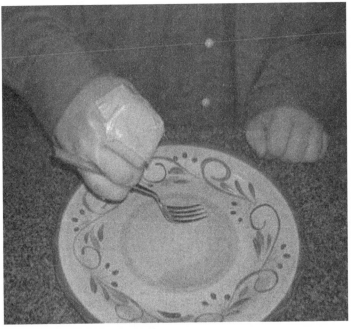

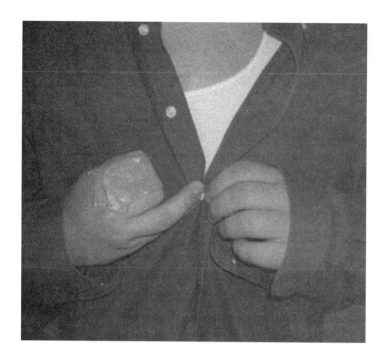

Along with underestimating the true value of fingers and the long-term consequences of hand injuries, most of us underestimate the time and agony of recovery. Days are missed. Weeks are missed. Recovery may require significant help from loved ones, drugs, lengthy physical therapy, multiple operations. Indeed, surgical repairs to the hand are notoriously difficult, and there's a high probability that a major injury will affect your dexterity forever.

As of this writing, the insurance industry estimates the value of a lost thumb or pointer finger at around $125,000, a whole lost hand at around $250,000;[9] but these are low numbers considering the limitations you would encounter for the rest of your life.

All for lack of the right PPE. Or a lack of attention. Or a lack of supervision.

OKAY, HERE'S A LIST

It's worth briefly listing some of the major hand injuries that occur in the workplace, just to show what you're up against.

- **Cuts:** Human skin is thin, and sharp edges are everywhere. That makes cuts the overwhelming number one on the list of hand injuries. Cuts can be minor or deep, cutting through ligaments, veins, or whole fingers.
- **Pinch points:** Tools and equipment create tight spaces that crush, twist, and tear whole hands. Especially moving machinery.
- **Lost fingers:** Common around rotating equipment and in food processing.
- **Impacts and crushings:** Tools, machinery, or materials smacking down, usually on the top of the hand: a major, if often-overlooked danger to working hands. Especially common in construction, as well as oil and gas work, where people are handling big wrenches, pipes, and equipment.
- **Abrasions:** Even if they don't catch a finger or a hand, moving parts like gears and lathes can abrade and tear at skin.
- **Repetitive injuries:** Repetitive tasks can cause injuries like carpal tunnel syndrome.
- **Heat:** Welding torches, foundry metals, plastics molding, and the hot moving parts of machines can burn deeply.
- **Cold** can cause frostbite.
- **Chemicals** can burn you immediately or cause serious conditions like cancer over long exposure. It's unbelievable how often workers are given the wrong gloves for the types of chemicals they are handling. This can include lubricating oils and metal-handling fluids of all kinds.
- **Electricity** can kill.

- **Vibration:** One common injury often overlooked by safety managers is hand-arm vibration syndrome (HAVS), a condition that affects hands working with pneumatic tools like jackhammers or vibrating machinery-like grinders. HAVS can cause neurological disorders, even vascular and skeletal problems. You get white fingers and you lose feeling.

Long-term effects are the most insidious: HAVS, carpal tunnel, and chemical exposures included. In training sessions, we will have workers hold some freshly cut garlic. After a time, they can taste the garlic in their mouths. Skin is porous, we tell them. It absorbs everything.

We also remind workers that hand injuries are often caused not by the task actually being done by the worker, but by the carelessness of others: tools left unsheathed, debris scattered in the area, machinery not locked out.

THE HUMAN FACTORS

Machines, chemicals, and tools are inherently dangerous. But human factors greatly increase the risk. These human factors operate at the level of the worker, the manager, and the organization at large—every level counts.

Indeed, it's rare that an injury is any one single person's fault.

A worker may lose focus on a task, and move a hand too close to a spinning lathe—we'll devote much discussion to the psychology of those moments. But a safety manager may also have failed to do an inspection that would have led to a barrier being placed to prevent that hand from *ever* moving too close.

Bad things happen to good hands because a worker has a lapse of attention, but also because the company has no safety manager.

Bad things happen to good hands because the company does no forward thinking about conditions and risks. Creates no accountability for injuries. Has no money for proper safety improvements. Succumbs to production pressures that move factory lines at unsafe speeds.

Bad things happen to good hands because an unwitting purchasing manager buys bulky, uncomfortable PPE that no one wears.

Bad things happen to good hands because a supervisor fails to set an example by wearing proper gloves, or setting safety guards on machinery. At some point, either verbally or through their body language, the manager has communicated, "Our protocols are a good idea, but they're optional."

Bad things happen to good hands because a supervisor thinks, "It's obvious how to do this safely. Anyone who puts their hand in the damn machine is stupid, and you can't fix stupid." *Actually, you can fix stupid. It's called training.*

Bad things happen to good hands because workers have lost trust and respect for management, do not believe that management cares, and no longer listen when managers set safety policies or run training sessions to improve safety.

Bad things happen to good hands because "safety training" consists of ten minutes on the worker's first (or fiftieth!) day, with no follow-up.

Bad things happen to good hands because safety trainers often have no experience with the actual work being done.

It all counts.

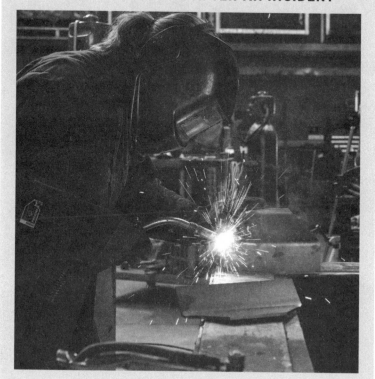

It's worth giving a careful read to this quote from a manager at an oil refinery parts manufacturer. What could have been done to prevent this accident from happening in the first place?

"Recently, one of our welders accidentally touched her hand with her TIG welding rod and burned a hole in her flesh, right through two pairs of gloves. She was wearing both leather TIG gloves *and* Kevlar gloves, but it went right through, and she had to have surgery to remove the cauterized flesh. The rod had just been welding, so it was probably at 1500° Fahrenheit and would have melted through any sort of synthetic product or leather.

"We've looked at the incident very carefully, and I don't think anything would have stopped it short of a piece of steel. A chainmail glove perhaps, but that's counterproductive for a welder, as they deal with electricity and heat all the time, and if you put something on them that's conductive to electricity and heat, it's not going to help. There's not much that would have stopped her getting injured other than not doing it in the first place.

"The incident came right at the end of the shift so the welder wasn't really focused. What she was doing was very repetitive, and she had become a little complacent. She was welding together some small parts that had to be turned over at some point—so rather than put the torch down and turn the part over and pick the torch up again, she just tried to flip it over while still holding the torch. That was very much something that she could have prevented.

"After the incident we gave all the welders a holder to put on their workstations. Now, rather than put a torch down on the bench and worry about it sliding off, they put it in this holder so it can't move."

Do you see? Sure, maybe the welder was tired at the end of the day—but she didn't put the torch down when she flipped the part over because there was no holder, and she was wor-

ried about it sliding off the table. Suppose the manager had watched the welders work and had discussed safety ideas with them once a month or even once a quarter to identify issues like this in advance of an incident? Suppose shift rotations had been shortened, as well?

NO THINKING-THROUGH OF SAFETY ISSUES

The single biggest human error contributing to hand injuries may simply be the tendency of humans to keep doing things the way they've been doing them for years, without stepping back to see the options, or reanalyze the work.

Or asking how times have changed.

For example, a local steel plant has been using the same leather glove for more than forty years. How do I know this? Because my father invented the glove for them around 1963. It was a great glove in its day, but far, far better options now exist—including highly cut-resistant Kevlar models that would be perfect for metalwork. Indeed, we've shown these guys dozens of better options, but they refuse to make the switch.

Why?

It's the glove they've always worn. They're used to it. It's like we're coming in and trying to switch out their brand of beer.

Safety takes proactive thought, planning, and engagement. The right solution is not always obvious and it takes an educated awareness of industry-specific issues.

Like I said, my company makes over 1,000 kinds of gloves. We make all those different kinds because sometimes you need a glove that gives cut protection, and sometimes you need crush protection, and sometimes you need both—and sometimes neither. Duh, right? But I can't tell you how many times I've seen companies buy cotton gloves for people using saws. Or people using cut-protective gloves to handle sharp metal while ignoring the fact that the metal is covered in a dangerous chemical that's soaking right through the Kevlar. Or people not using their big uncomfortable gloves because they're all padded up for crush protection, when there's no real danger of crushing.

Poor Accessibility

Or never mind all that. How many times have companies bought excellent gloves that just stay in the boxes because nobody enforces usage of the gloves? Or because the gloves are stored somewhere across the plant where they're hard to find and get at?

In manufacturing, construction, oil and gas, utility work—you name it—it takes a whole lot of planning to make sure you have the right thing in the right place at the right time.

I remember some construction workers on a highrise telling me how often a worker would get to the top of a building they were working on only to realize they didn't have their gloves with them. They'd look down, and there's a big locker full of gloves, way at the bottom of the structure. Do they bother to go back down and up, a journey of twenty minutes each way? Or do they just shrug and start work?

Who's doing the forward thinking to make sure this doesn't happen?

Penny-Pinching

In one sports equipment manufacturing plant I visited, the workers had to go to the safety manager and request a new pair of gloves when needed, knowing they'd get a hard time: "Why do you need new gloves? What happened to your last pair?" the safety manager would ask, just like the worker was a kid who'd lost their mittens. No doubt the manager was told to stay within the glove-purchasing budget and control costs. Maybe he saved a couple hundred bucks a year this way. Naturally, the workers kept wearing gloves with holes in them, and worked without gloves when one got lost. They didn't want the hassle or the lecture.

As a result of this apparently trivial, small-thinking policy, hands were maimed and injured.

Indeed, a few years later, when upper management figured out what was happening to their worker's comp insurance, they put out big barrels of gloves, so people could just grab them when needed. They worried a bit about pilfering, but figured they could lose a whole lot of gloves, and still come out ahead, not just health-wise and morale-wise, but money-wise.

Indeed, in my work, I see this happen again and again. Often it's only upper management who can really see how safety contributes to the bottom line, because they're the ones who see the ultimate costs of injuries, lost time, and all the other real costs of penny-pinching.

SAFETY TRAINING AFTER THE FACT

A story from a colleague of mine, let's call her Linda: "I got a new job at a big agribusiness chemical concern, calibrating automated machinery for pesticide delivery on crops in different provinces. My first day on the job," says Linda, "I was flown across the country, and when I arrived, I received the keys for my vehicle. Just like that, boom, I headed out on my own. That same afternoon, I started working with incredibly dangerous fungicides, pesticides, and other chemicals, and doing these calibrations of equipment. About four months in, I got an email telling me to come to headquarters for my safety training. That email was so funny, I laughed out loud."

Worker Attitudes, Worker Culture, and Cognitive Biases

In chapter three we're going to dive deep into the crucial issue of safety psychology, but I've put worker attitudes, worker culture, and cognitive biases at the end of my list of human factors for a reason. Safety starts with the attitude of management, not the attitude of workers. And safety is ultimately the responsibility of management, too. No getting around it.

That said, the mindset of the worker *in the moment* matters enormously when it comes to hand safety.

Bad things happen to good hands because tools are used improperly—even though workers were trained on how to use them properly.

Bad things happen because safety mechanisms are disabled in a moment of frustration, in order to get something done quicker. Or because "I just need to do this one thing."

Bad things happen because sometimes workers come from a culture where fatalism is rampant or where people accept injuries as an inevitable fact of life. In these cultures, people may say, "There's nothing you can do about it. Accidents just happen. It's all in the hands of God."

SOME QUOTES FROM SAFETY MANAGERS

"Probably 80 percent of these guys think it's a good idea to put on all their PPE...There is a portion of the guys that feel it is just a pain in the ass and we will do it because we have to but we don't really need to do that."

"When the safety people are around everybody is doing things right, and when they leave it goes back to not using PPE."

"They tend to take shortcuts—'It's not going to happen to me today'...They tend to push the envelope."

"Most of the drivers buy into [using PPE]...but sometimes they are apathetic, they get sloppy and they cut corners, and it's just human nature."

Bad things happen because workers become careless with the safety of others, such as in leaving debris or dangerous tools lying around unprotected—a box cutter left open on a worktable, for example.

Bad things happen because workers ignore policies and procedures.

Bad things happen because workers don't say anything when they see a hazard.

Bad things happen to good hands because people keep going even when they know they're too tired to be safe.

THE UNSEEN DANGER

In addition to all the above, every human is subject to cognitive biases which impair their ability to see and react to dangers.

Safety expert, Matt Hallowell, offers the perfect example. He says to imagine a crew drilling into the earth with two big, powered augers.[10] One is spinning and one is not. It's obvious the spinning auger is dangerous and everyone stays back. But the one that's *not* spinning may be the more dangerous. Maybe it's stuck, and enormous forces are building up and it's about to break apart and go flying in all directions.

An experienced worker would immediately spot this danger, right? Maybe. Ironically, experienced workers can sometimes be even more at risk to unseen dangers than inexperienced workers, because they are not looking at a situation with fresh eyes. A safety manager for oil rigs once told me that he visited an offshore platform and was going through his checklist when he asked, "Where are the lifeboats?" No one knew the answer, even the guys who had been working out there for years. A new worker coming onto the rig? Lifeboats might be his first question.

We'll explore plenty of other cognitive biases that threaten workers in chapter three.

THINGS THAT HAPPEN

Here's a story from a municipal utility worker doing sewer line construction. "Last week we were out in what we call our TV truck, which runs cameras down the tunnels with long cables, to do inspections. The cable reel has big, dangerous gears which are supposed to have protective guards covering them. But the guys had removed these guards to adjust something, and they didn't bother to put them back on when they started the reel back up. I guess they were just in a hurry. So one guy caught the tip of his finger, and the gears cut it right off. He was wearing gloves, but the gloves didn't help."

At a poultry processing facility, a worker was trying to unclog a chicken marinade pump. He removed the hose that was secured with a clamp and stuck his finger in, where it was lobbed off by the impeller.[11] Just dumb? Maybe no one told him to shut off the machines before trying a fix? Maybe they figured "anyone would know that?"

At a beef processing plant, a worker cutting a carcass with a saw took off his own fingers.[12] Chainmail gloves might have saved him, but he had none on. Were they unavailable? Did he just get careless?

At a tire processing plant in Canada, a kid was pulled into a tire shredding machine and died.[13] It had no emergency stop button. Imagine a tire shredding machine with no emergency stop button!

At an auto insulation factory in Ohio, a worker got his hand caught in a waste shredding machine while he was guiding waste into it. Part of his forearm had to be amputated. No guard mechanism was on the machine to prevent this from happening. The machine had been used for years without incident—but without the guard, this specific incident was always waiting to happen. The government fined the factory $570,000.[14]

There's a rule of thumb (bad pun) that you shouldn't wear gloves while operating rotating equipment, because the machinery can grab the glove and take the skin off your hand with it, an event known euphemistically as being "degloved." A sixty-three-year-old man, nearing retirement, had worked as a machine engineer at a company for most of his life. He was extremely experienced with a machine that included a flywheel to drive the mechanism—maybe too experienced. It was his habit to wear gloves to slow down the flywheel when necessary, and he wore a driver's-style, loose-fit leather glove for that purpose. But this time, for some reason, his hand strayed to the choke, allowing the spinning wheel to grab the glove and snatch it off, along with three of his fingers.[15] Could training have prevented this? Some kind of guard? Certainly something more than experience was required; the way he'd been working had *always* been dangerously wrong, for decades.

Safety expert, Sam Cunard, tells the story of a construction worker in California who cut his hand because he was wearing gloves with no cut protection.[16] The little cut was apparently no big deal, so he didn't report it. Or treat it. Turns out he got a tiny splinter down deep inside, undetected, so the little cut never healed. Eventually, the cut got infected with MRSA. Eventually, the entire hand had to be amputated. Could better gloves, along with mandatory injury reporting have saved his hand?

Well, probably yes.

THINGS HAPPEN BECAUSE OF OVERALL COMPANY CULTURE

All of the above hand injuries were preventable. Indeed, the vast majority of hand injuries are preventable. They just are. If they're not prevented, it's symptomatic of something wrong with a company's overall culture. No forethought. No policies. Policies not enforced. Inadequate training. Bad attitudes. Workers getting fatalistic.

Importantly, attitude is not an individual event. Attitude is a shared experience that starts at the top. At a good company, the safety culture is so strong that in order to be part of the popular, insider "gang," you have to be safe. At a bad company, safety is not even discussed—it's practically a taboo subject, as if by mentioning safety concerns you were going to bring on the gaze of a fatalistic, evil eye.

In fact, fatalism is probably the leading indicator of a bad company. At a bad company, you will find a pervasive, ingrained attitude that some injuries are just inevitable. They're an unavoidable cost of operation, same as the cost of supplies. Same as the cost of (interchangeable) labor. Same as the inevitable safety fines. Among workers, the same fatalism will take hold—bad stuff is going to happen if it's your unlucky day. No avoiding it.

Let me put a stake in the ground. Fatalism is *immoral* both at the management level *and* at the worker level. That's because fatalism is an abdication of responsibility. It's never "all in God's hands."

At a good company, not only is fatalism completely rejected, they believe in trying to get to *zero injuries.* They believe it's *possible.* Even more, they believe that zero injuries make for good ROI. They know that not only will zero injuries mean that worker's comp costs go down and safety fines will disappear, but workers will have improved productivity as their trust increases. Retention will shoot up, because caring is a two-way street.

Let me end this chapter about "why bad things happen to good hands" with a story about one of my salespeople visiting a large, well-known brewery. He asked the COO how many hand injuries they had on a typical day, and the COO said, "Something like ten or twelve." My salesman, trying to make nice, said, "I guess that's not too big a deal, since you have about 500 employees working onsite on a typical day."

The COO got angry.

He said, "No, that is a very big deal, not just because people are getting hurt, but because I lose five or six hours every day for injuries. Even if they just get a little cut, they have to stop and go get first aid. They have to fill out some forms. It's a minimum of half an hour before they're back at work, and sometimes they're out for days. Ten or twelve injuries a day is a very, very big deal. That's why I have you standing here to talk about better gloves!"

That COO was starting to see the big picture.

He was starting to see that when bad things happen to good hands, everyone suffers.

And he was ready to take action.

CHAPTER TWO

THE TOP TEN HAND SAFETY MISTAKES

Now that we've seen why bad things happen to good hands, and why *all i*njuries reflect the overall culture of an organization, let's bring that information together into a top ten of bad approaches to safety. I figure if I boil it down to ten, the list will focus our minds for the chapters to come.

I'm tempted to imitate the late-night talk show hosts, and do my countdown from ten to one, with a big dramatic drumroll for number one. But number one is too important to bury like that. If a company gets number one wrong, each of the other mistakes will *inevitably follow.*

So let's just go right there.

MISTAKE #1: THINKING SAFETY IS A LINE RESPONSIBILITY INSTEAD OF A TOP MANAGEMENT RESPONSIBILITY

Way too often, the people sitting in conference rooms at the tops of office towers have *absolutely no idea if their workers are safe*. Much less any idea *how to keep them safe*.

Way too often, the people at the tops of office towers think of safety as some kind of regulatory checkbox or housekeeping item—something you delegate down to the warehouse supervisor, or the yard boss, or the shop foreman, or the ship's captain, or the crew lead out at the site.

Many top managers go further and assume that even supervisors cannot control safety. They believe that safety comes only from "worker attitudes" the company cannot influence. They say things like, "Those guys are a tough bunch doing a tough job, and they're gonna do what they're gonna do."

But here's the deal: without safety leadership coming from the very top of the office tower, from the boardroom and the CEO's office, no company will *ever* develop a genuine culture of safety. Without direction from the top, you will *never* see safety thinking at every level of a company, or a true spirit of team safety, or consistently good decisions made right down to the level of the guy or gal operating the pneumatic drill.

Not only do I never see downstream safety thinking without upstream safety thinking, I know it's impossible.

Partly that's because workers derive their personal attitudes very much from company attitudes. In later chapters, we'll look more closely at how and why that happens, but for now let's just say that *people usually decide what to care about based on what the boss cares about.*

If the boss doesn't care enough about safety, right on up to the top boss, neither will most of the people down the line. In the sidebar, ex-CEO Paul O'Neill talks about the way he had to shock his managers into taking personal responsibility for safety at Alcoa. I love this example, because it illustrates how leadership matters, and how sometimes a leader has to shock the troops.

"WE KILLED HIM"

This is from a speech Paul O'Neill, ex-CEO of Alcoa, gave about management taking the responsibility for safety.

"Oftentimes, the things that move organizations are, unfortunately, not happy stories. But after I'd been [at Alcoa] about three months...there was an incident at an extrusion plant outside of Phoenix, Arizona. This was a night shift. There was an eighteen-year-old kid who'd worked for the company for about three weeks. He jumped over a protective barrier... between his observation space and the machine that was producing extrusions. This particular machine had a boom on it, so with every cycle the boom would cycle, cycle, cycle. The machine was subject to jamming. The aluminum material would get jammed in the machine and it would be hung up. This kid jumped over the barrier and pulled the scrap material out of the action part of the machine and it released the boom. It came around and hit him in the head. Killed him instantly. He had a wife who was six months pregnant.

"Two supervisors who had been there fifteen or twenty years watched him do it. Actually, they must have taught him how to do it, because I don't think he made it up on his own to jump over the barrier and pull the material out of the machine.

"So I got the whole executive crowd together, all the way down to the plant supervisor level. We reviewed the diagrams and the machine process and all of that. When we were done with that technical part, I stood up and said to the assembled crowd, 'We killed him. Yeah, the supervisors were there, but we killed him. I killed him, because I didn't do a good job of communicating the dedication to the principle that people will *never* be hurt at work. Obviously, our recruiting process didn't do a very good job or our measurement process didn't do a very good job of assuring that people who are in this chain believed that safety was the single most important thing.'

"...I tell you what, the people in the organization were stunned by the idea that they should accept personal responsibility for this death. [Sure,] they all *regretted* it. I tell you, there was never a more caring organization in my experience, in a traditional sense, than Alcoa. Every person that was injured or killed, they *mourned.* Believe me, they really mourned them. They regretted it and all of that, but [until then] they didn't understand they *were responsible* for it."[17]

MISTAKE #2: LOOKING AT SAFETY AS AN *ADDITIONAL COST*

How many companies put up signs that say "safety first" at their plants?

How many companies will insert the words "our people are our most important asset" into every single after-dinner speech given by every company officer?

Now, where's the proof that those words have meaning?

As I mentioned in the introduction, when Paul O'Neill took over Alcoa in 1987, he told the investment community, "If you want to know how Alcoa is doing, look at our safety record." To many, it was a bizarre and troubling statement, and it sent the stock tumbling.

As a colleague put it, "Every time he talked, his first words out of his mouth were about safety. Every meeting, the first agenda item was safety...[Alcoa] had 28 businesses and they would come in quarterly for a review with the CEO. The first item they were expected to cover was safety. It wasn't finances. It was safety. Now, of course they covered their finances and they covered market share and they covered everything else, but the first item was always safety..."[18]

O'Neill believed that focusing on safety would improve the overall success of the company over time, and he was right. Within a year of his astounding speech about safety, Alcoa's profits would hit a record high. By the time he retired in 2000, the company's annual net income was five times higher than when he arrived. Meanwhile, the company's lost day worker injury rate fell to one-twentieth the US average.[19]

When he was installed as CEO, Alcoa's lost time injury rate was 1.86.[20] By the time he retired, it was down to 0.2. By 2012, it had continued to drop, to 0.125. Indeed, when he took over, O'Neill announced that he wanted that injury rate to drop to *zero*. He described the reaction of his board and lieutenants like this:

"[They said] we can't afford it. In order to really get to zero we're going to have to wrap every employee in some kind of a cocoon and they won't be able to move their arms to do the work. We can't afford it."

O'Neill's response was that safety should not be a budget item *at all.* "Safety should never be a priority," he said, "it should be a precondition. Like, before you can get up and walk around, you have to breathe. Safety should be like breathing. It should be a precondition for organizational behavior."

Once you start "budgeting for safety," once you start thinking about safety as a "cost" in your ledger, once you say "here's how much safety we can afford" or "here's the injury rate that's reasonable within our cost structure," you have already lost sight of *safety first.* You have already proven that your people are not your most *important asset.*

And believe me, your people notice. If you don't make their safety your highest priority, your people will not make your company's success their highest priority. They will not do their best work. The sense of order and responsibility necessary to any great manufacturing, construction, food, oil and gas, aerospace, or other hands-on concern will be lost. The opposite is also true:

"To the extent that you develop real excellence in safety, you will also create a high performance culture, which will improve your effectiveness and efficiency in general."

—THOMAS KRAUSE[21]

Put even more simply: putting safety first works not just for people, but for the bottom line.

"YOU ARE AN IDIOT!"

Need more evidence that safety offers a high ROI? Big companies tend to have far better safety records than small companies. Among manufacturing firms, for example, the fatality rate is nearly eight times higher for the smallest establishments (1–19 workers) than for big establishments (1,000+ workers). The smallest establishments have more than three times the fatalities than the next size up (20-49 workers).[22]

Why is that? Well, big companies do tend to offer all the infrastructure of safety managers, training, and oversight. But just as importantly, they have professional company management that does ROI analyses!

Some years ago, I was working with a major aerospace company, helping them pick out the right gloves for some of their manufacturing workers. We had done trials and convinced the line managers to go from a general purpose glove to a cut-resistant glove. We had lots of trial data which absolutely, conclusively showed, "This will significantly reduce your hand injuries."

The change was enthusiastically approved by the line managers, but then somebody in accounting sent an email that said, "No, there's no way we're going from $1 glove to an $8 glove. That's not happening!"

Heated meetings were held between the line managers and the accounting guys until at last the CEO called the accounting guy and said, in so many words, "Approve the damn PO 'cause we're gonna save about a million dollars a year on injuries! You wanna save $50,000 in gloves? You are an idiot because you are exactly being 'penny wise and pound foolish!'"

The gloves were approved. Injuries went down. And indeed, the company saved millions. Oh, and people's hands, too.

Need an overall ROI calculator for safety and glove costs? See the appendix or www.rethinkinghandsafety.com.

MISTAKE #3: THINKING SOME ACCIDENTS ARE INEVITABLE

At the end of chapter two I talked about the evils of fatalism. Let's go just a little deeper. In fact, let's start with a statement you may consider controversial, but I consider vital:

> You must always work from an assumption that you can get your company to zero injuries.

How could that possibly be true? The minute you admit that some rate of injury is inevitable, you are subscribing to fatalism of one kind or another. This fatalism *can and will* be communicated in both subtle and not so subtle ways.

If you shrug when you say, "These guys come from a culture where injuries are just taken for granted," you are yourself being fatalistic and reinforcing whatever fatalism occurs among your workforce.

If you are a shift supervisor and you walk into the workplace without wearing PPE, you are not just saying that PPE is unimportant, you are not just saying you don't care if your workers wear their PPE, you are saying that "some level of injury is unavoidable, so why try?"

If you do not make an effort to understand what is being done at other companies in your same industry to reduce injuries, you are saying that your company is somehow different, and somehow "less fixable" than your competitors.

If you ever once say to a coworker, "Nothing could have been done to prevent that" you are crippling future preventive measures. If you ever once say, "Humans are imperfect, so bad stuff will happen" you are ensuring the next round of bad stuff. If you ever once say, "We did all we could," you are subscribing to no-responsibility fatalism. Indeed, you are establishing fatalism as the norm. You are dooming the safety initiatives both in your time and in future times at your company.

If you are a safety manager, or a supervisor, or anyone in authority, you must *always, and in all circumstances* say that the *only* acceptable number of injuries is zero injuries. Full stop.

MISTAKE #4: USING MISGUIDED SAFETY INCENTIVES

One day a company official stands up at a board meeting and says, "We want to create a safer environment and improve our safety record, right? Let's offer a bonus to any work crew that goes three months injury-free! Then we'll take them all out for pizza!"

To the ignorant, this may seem like a logical and positive step. But it's a bad idea. A very bad idea. Even illegal in some contexts.

You see, research has proven again and again that such incentives lead to the *covering-up* of injuries, rather than the reduction of injuries. Managers and even workers will simply stop reporting incidents so as not to break their streak, or to improve their quarterly numbers and win a prize. That means workers don't get the proper care. That means that proper reporting to government agencies doesn't occur.

At one company, for example, a pregnant woman told a researcher that she'd fallen on the job one day, but her team actually told her not to go to the doctor because it would "create too much paperwork and ruin our numbers."

You get a streak of non-reporting, not a streak of no injuries.

Even worse are penalties for supervisors or work teams that show high rates of injuries. One study run with union carpenters, for example, found that injury reporting dropped by 50 percent when workers were either penalized or disciplined for high numbers—while the actual rate of injuries stayed the same.[23]

Psychologically and culturally, such incentives or penalties also tend to shift responsibility and blame from management to workers, by saying, in effect, "If you were only behaving properly, you wouldn't get hurt." No matter how well-intentioned, the wrong incentives create bad feelings.

Want to create useful incentives? Think about rewarding positive efforts made to create safe conditions. You can reward people for great ideas to improve safety. You can reward people for wearing their gloves every day. You can reward supervisors for giving regular safety training sessions. You can reward workers for attending safety training sessions.

Such incentives say, "We're on your side."

WHAT ABOUT PENALTIES?

Any kind of penalties, even for unsafe behaviors, must be thought through with substantial care. Individual workers might be cautioned, then warned, then even fired for not wearing their gloves on the job. Supervisors can be cautioned, warned, then fired for not enforcing specific safety policies—but again, not for their statistics.

What about public shaming? Only with great caution. For example, at one construction company, workers who forgot their assigned gloves were forced to wear bright pink gloves provided by the work supervisor. Because of the general sense of camaraderie and gentle ribbing in this particular crew, the policy seemed to work, and it got positive reviews from workers. But in another company, depending on the cultural context, such a tactic might backfire. It might seem patronizing and disrespectful—as if hand safety were not a life and death issue.

We'll talk more about incentives and punishments in chapter four, where we discuss company culture.

MISTAKE #5: SAYING YOU CAN'T FIX STUPID

Up on the wall of a manufacturing plant in a city I won't name there's a sign which shows a photo of a man's hand with several fingers cut off. Underneath this picture, it says, "Steve wasn't listening. Steve cut his fingers off. Don't be Steve."

Let's think about this sign for a moment. Whoever posted it was trying to be shocking, funny, and memorable, all at the same time.

But what that sign really says is this: "If you get injured, it's because you're stupid." Beyond that, it says, "This is the best that we, management, can do to protect you. No training, no PPE, no policies will fix your stupidity." Finally, the sign has zero respect for the pain and suffering of "Steve."

Overall, this sign implies a vast gulf between the person who posted the sign and the workers who are reading it, as in: "We're fundamentally different, you workers and we management types. I have to talk down to you or you won't listen. And I have the right to post pictures of, like, your injuries. *We're not on the same team, you and me.*"

Ultimately, a sign like this is *counterproductive to* safe behaviors. Why? Because no one thinks they themselves are stupid. They will pass that sign and think, "Well, that could happen to an idiot, but it won't happen to me, because I'm not an idiot." So they don't take the proper precautions that anyone, smart or stupid, should take.

Believe me, the workers in that plant do not think that sign is funny. Only their managers think it's funny.

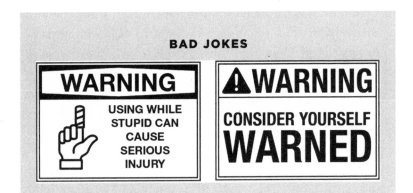

BAD JOKES

Here are two truly awful safety signs from the same manufacturing plant. Imagine if you worked beneath one of these signs, or actually incurred an injury at a machine it was posted above. You would hate the management which put up these "jokes."

The second sign, about being warned, actually reinforces the message of the first, and implies the general stupidity of workers. Like the first, it says, "We're not even going to bother giving you specific instructions on how to be safe in this environment, because it should be obvious to anyone with common intelligence."

Again and again, in manufacturing plants, out on oil rigs, or riding on utility trucks, you will hear the refrain, "You can't fix stupid." As if, no matter what safety precautions are taken, people are ultimately responsible for their own safety, and if they do stupid things, they'll get stupid injuries.

This is a dangerous, even an unforgivable attitude. As in Mistake #3, it means that you are assuming that some injuries are inevitable, and you are ignoring the chain of responsibility which leads to *all* injuries, which are *never* just one person's fault.

Maybe Steve didn't put the guard down on a table saw before he used it. But maybe the guard was poorly designed and interfered with the work, so everyone tended to leave it up. Maybe the guard was broken off, and hadn't been replaced. Maybe there'd been no training on how to use the table saw safely before Steve started working on it. Maybe Steve wasn't wearing his cut-resistant gloves because they were hot and bulky and uncomfortable, having been purchased by some purchasing agent who never had the people on the floor actually try them out first.

MISTAKE #6: FORGETTING YOUR WORKERS SPEAK DIFFERENT LANGUAGES

I can't tell you how often I've been in factories or out on construction sites where *most* of the workers speak little or no English, but *all* the safety signs and *all* the safety training are only in English.

Really, it's kind of incredible.

A manager once actually said to me, "Well, if they want to work here, they need to learn English *eventually,*" as if until they learned better English, they were somehow expendable. As if this worker were not putting his or her life on the line *today* for this manager.

In another company we visited, 90 percent of the workforce was Filipino and spoke Tagalog as their mother tongue, but all the signs and training were English-only. When we gently inquired about this, the CEO told us, "Our company only works in English. All our clients speak English. We speak English. We're an English-speaking company."

Okay, fair enough for your business relationships, even with your workers. *But for safety?*

One study conducted in New Orleans found that 57 percent of Latino construction workers, for example, received *no* safety training.[24] Notice that I didn't say "Spanish-speaking." That's because plenty of Latino workers don't necessarily speak good Spanish, either. They may speak an indigenous dialect, with only limited Spanish—though no one may have bothered to inquire. You could probably extrapolate this study to much of the construction industry in the US.

THE DANGER OF NODDING AND SMILING

Immigrants with poor language skills may nod and smile at training classes, or when told a safety policy, even though they've not understood a word. You've probably done something like that yourself when visiting a foreign country.

Ensuring the safety of multilingual workers does take time, effort, education, and additional money. Ignorant and half-hearted efforts may be useless. For example, I've seen plenty of signs with complicated instructions in English, supplemented by a simple, "international diagram" that conveys little of the full information.

Suppose you went to work in Sweden with only a poor command of Swedish. One day you are confronted with a complicated and dangerous machine. Above the machine is a sign with three paragraphs in Swedish, but only one pictogram with a guy's hand X-ed out. Translation: *Good luck, buddy.*

When that sign was pointed out, you might just nod and smile, so no one knew you couldn't read the language of your bosses.

MISTAKE #7: IGNORING CULTURAL ISSUES

We need to talk more about immigrants. Why? Because in the most dangerous professions in all countries, a high proportion of the workers facing that danger are often from other countries. That's just the way the world operates.[25]

This situation leads to more than mismatches of language, it leads to dangerous mismatches of culture.

People from other countries often have very different cultures when it comes to health and safety. It's your job not to ignore those differences.

Immigrants may be from war-torn countries where something like a gashed hand just isn't considered that big a deal: "Hey, no one's getting bombed or shot, so why wear all this PPE? This construction site is the safest place I ever worked."

Immigrants may have been raised in a culture with a powerful machismo which makes them think wearing gloves implies weakness or a lack of courage. Or that telling others about your pain shows a lack of toughness.

Immigrants may have been raised in a culture where you just never say you don't know something or don't know how to do something—where to admit ignorance would be to lose face. As pointed out in Mistake #6, they may also be pretending they speak English better than they do. They may be pretending they understood that training on tag-out and lock-out, when they never understood a word.

But be aware that this pretending may also have deep cultural roots, beyond just trying to make their way in a foreign country.

Indeed, immigrants may have been raised in a culture with a truly enormous class difference between management and workers, where workers just keep their problems among themselves, and never talk to a manager if it can be avoided. They may automatically keep quiet about health and safety dangers which they and their fellows face daily.

Immigrants may be from countries that practice folk medicine or follow archaic ideas about health and safety that conflict with modern logic. For example, some agricultural workers may not wash their hands in cold water on a hot day, even though they are covered in pesticides. Why? They practice a humoral medicine which teaches that mixing hot and cold causes illness.[26]

Immigrants may come from a culture with a heavily fatalistic view of injuries, as in, "If it's your day to get hurt, you are just going to get hurt, and nothing can protect you. That's how God and the universe work."

You will have to work directly against that view of the universe, because you are a *safety manager*.

CAUTIOUS ABOUT THEIR STATUS

The issue of an immigrant's status will also get in the way. Even if they have all their papers, they rightly feel less certain of their position in society.

You may have a policy that all injuries must be reported immediately, but an immigrant may not want to report a gash on their hand because it might make them look stupid or clumsy or a complainer—and if they were to lose their job, the consequences of that loss might be far higher than for other workers. Far worse than shutting up, wrapping the hand, and continuing work. If they're in your country without legal documentation, the consequences may be extreme, indeed.

Once again, it's your job to protect people, no matter what their personal circumstances. That means making them comfortable reporting injuries, unsafe conditions, and unease about the safety of certain tasks.

PEOPLE JUST DON'T THINK THE SAME

Bottom line: we tend to think that other people think the same as we do and will act as we do, but we are often wrong. Indeed, it's far more difficult just to interpret the facial expressions of people from other cultures. Are they happy? Sad? Angry? These expressions, or sometimes purposeful lack of expression, are often culturally rooted, and not universal at all.

Study after study shows the danger of being an immigrant worker anywhere. In the US, for example, a study of 7,000 construction workers found that Hispanic workers are 30 percent more likely to have medical conditions due to work-related injuries than non-Hispanics.[27] Why? Well, see all of the above, starting with the language barriers we discussed in Mistake #6.

MANAGEMENT'S FATALISM ABOUT IMMIGRANTS

One last thing about cultural issues. One of the biggest dangers faced by immigrants to any country from any other country may be the fatalistic attitude that *management* often has about their injuries.

Management may have a stated or unstated attitude that says: "Oh, yeah, those guys are going to get hurt, they just do."

Management may even consciously or subconsciously think that migrants are somehow expendable, because "more will be coming along soon."

It happens. It's also morally wrong.

MISTAKE #8: BAD PPE BUYING AND STORING HABITS

We once visited a metal shelving manufacturer—extremely dangerous work, with employees handling sharp edges every minute of the day. The company bought a lot of gloves because gloves got shredded, and quickly. Since they bought so many gloves, they looked for the cheapest leather models they could, like $1 a pair in bulk.

Naturally, their workers' hands were getting shredded too. So much so that the company employed a full-time nurse just to stitch people up. We went in to talk to the purchasing manager and said, "Hey, we've got a glove that would certainly reduce your injuries by 90 percent. Not 80 percent, 90 percent. It's highly cut-resistant, and it's flexible too." These new gloves probably cost four times what the old ones cost, per pair. About $4 instead of $1, so yes, it would be an investment.

The purchasing guy flat out replied, "We could never afford those gloves."

"But along with so many fewer injuries, the company would end up saving money in the long run," we protested. "Less nursing time. Lower worker's comp insurance. Less time off work. "

"Sure," replied the purchasing guy, "But that's a different budget. There's no way I can allocate more money for gloves." And that was that. The company ended up staying with the cheap gloves and keeping the nurse.

The nurse probably cost them upwards of $60,000 a year. But she was on someone else's budget.

DOES THE PURCHASING DEPT DETERMINE SAFETY?

Don't get me wrong, I love purchasing managers. *But no one should be allowed to select personal protective equipment who does not have direct experience with the work.* No one should be allowed to select PPE who's unwilling to do a genuine job hazard assessment to see what's actually needed.

It's absolutely astonishing to me that a company executive who has never spoken to a worker about the actual work being done could say, "Let's buy these gloves, they're probably good enough." Or, "Let's buy these sleeves. Or aprons. Or helmets. Or whatever. They look fine."

But it happens every day.

Purchasing managers may err in the opposite direction, by the way. They may buy gloves that are unnecessarily bulky for the work. Or get too hot and sweaty. Or offer great cut resistance, but no protection from the cold. So the expensive new gloves don't get used.

As a result of this bad choice, out on the actual oil derrick or road repair truck or top of a skyscraper, men and women are going dangerously bare-handed. *And the purchasing manager never even knows.*

The heavy, bulky, expensive, unused gloves may have been chosen to cover management's ass. The purchasing manager may have thought, "We'll get the maximum protection, and then no one can ever complain that we didn't do our best!" He or she may even have said that in a boardroom.

3M corporation once did a study[28] where they asked workers if they knew why they were wearing certain PPE, and plenty said they didn't really know, they just knew they were supposed to wear these heavy gloves or this hearing protection—but no one had actually explained the hazard or how the PPE related to it. In essence, they assumed the company was just covering its ass.

Like I said, my company makes 1,000 different kinds of gloves for a reason. Never done a hazard assessment? See chapter seven of this book. Need to learn the rules of glove buying? See chapter six.

DISTRUST BREEDS DISTRUST

Of course, sometimes the problem goes deeper than letting the purchasing department drive safety decisions.

Sometimes companies buy the cheapest PPE because they simply don't trust their employees. They think their employees might steal expensive gloves or other equipment and take the stuff home. They think, "Let them steal the $1 gloves, not the $10 kind."

That kind of distrust is contagious. The employees catch it, too. They stop believing you care, so they stop listening to your hollow pronouncements about safety. They stop paying attention to your safety training and safety policies, so everyone gets less safe.

LETTING BOB PICK HIS OWN GLOVE

As I pointed out in chapter two, the exact inverse of the purchasing manager problem comes when companies allow employees to pick whatever glove they want, willy nilly, as in:

Hey, Bob likes that kind of glove. We love Bob, so get that glove for Bob!

In that kind of company, everyone's wearing a different glove—and we've seen literally 300 different kinds of gloves in a single facility, among people doing the *same job*. This is almost as bad as the choice from the ignorant purchasing department, because individual workers often don't know what's the best kind of glove for their work, have no knowledge of what's available, and have never done their own systematic hazard analysis.

Often as not, they'll pick a glove for comfort, not real protection. And they'll take it from one kind of task over to do a completely different kind of task the next day.

Bob may be real happy…until he loses a finger.

We'll talk more about how to choose gloves in chapter six.

LOCKING THE GOOD STUFF AWAY

At this point, I have to mention a curious problem I've seen even at companies that actually do the right thing in purchasing PPE.

They've done their hazard assessment; they've spent the right money for the right equipment. *So now they take extra special care of that expensive PPE by locking it carefully away on the far side of the plant.* Management makes workers sign out for the good stuff on a daily basis. They give workers a hard time when stuff gets lost or needs replacing.

As a result, people are less safe, not more safe because of the purchase.

If someone has to walk a quarter mile to get new gloves or new hearing protection or whatever, they're just not going to do it all the times they need to do it. PPE has to be close by. It has to be convenient.

Not five minutes away, but five seconds away. With no hassle.

Yes, good PPE is valuable, but uh…only if it's used.

MISTAKE #9: SETTLING FOR LOUSY TRAINING AND DULL TRAINERS

The state of safety training in the industry is surprisingly abysmal. Often it's just a checkbox for management, without any real thought going into the process. As a result, much training fails to produce any results, and the trainers don't seem to realize why it has failed. "These workers are just dumb," they say later. "They just don't listen."

But guess what? If workers aren't listening to your training, it's your failure, not theirs.

Training is often generic, without workers being consulted about the actual dangers they face.

Training is often boring, with little thought given on how to engage workers.

Training is often one-way, with no discussion or input from listeners during a lecture.

Training often consists just of words, without demonstrations or hands-on experiences to develop "muscle memory" for safety.

People who work with their hands are a kind of athlete. Athletes don't just train from PowerPoint shows.

Training is often dumbed down in an insulting way. When you treat workers like children, they stop listening.

I have a whole chapter on training, later on, but here's a clue: Adults learn best when you present the problem, before giving the solution to the problem. That means they need to hear the logic behind a policy, not just the policy itself. They also need to believe that you have considered multiple alternatives, just as they would themselves before they settled on the right approach. You need to say things like:

"We tried that solution, but it didn't work, so the policy is this."

Unfortunately, much training consists of nothing more than, "Here's a bullet list of do's and don'ts."

CREDIBILITY COUNTS...A LOT

Perhaps most importantly, safety training is often performed by people who have no credibility with the workers.

Nothing tunes people out faster than an instructor who shows that he or she does not understand the real hazards faced by real workers out in their real environment.

Real example: An outside trainer was brought into a factory to show workers how they should safely carry heavy loads. He spent a half-hour showing how to lift and carry, including, "Make sure to carry the weight close to your body." When he said that, people actually laughed out loud. Why? Much of their work included carrying around caustic chemicals in buckets. The last thing they would ever do would be to carry those buckets close to their bodies. Result? *Loss of credibility for all future training performed by the company.*[29]

BUT CREDIBILITY CAN BE MISUSED

Of course, boring trainers can come in all shapes and sizes and experience levels. Sometimes, even their working credibility can work *against* your goals. Someone who has been doing the work for thirty years and knows all the issues may be terrible at speaking to a group, may be way behind on current safety techniques, and may scoff at company regulations.

One skeptical raise of the eyebrows at a company policy by an experienced worker (or worse, a supervisor) doing training may undo everything in your carefully constructed PowerPoint show.

Read the training chapter in this book. In fact, read it two or three times. I talked to some real artists in the field to create that chapter, and in the course of those conversations, I learned that safety training, like all teaching, is less science than art. But no art has ever been more vital to humans.

MISTAKE #10: KEEPING USELESS STATS

Probably you keep statistics on your annual rates of injury. On average you had, say twelve per month this year, and fourteen per month last year. You have a bar graph showing your OSHA Recordable Total Incident Rate dropping from 1.87 to 1.73 per one hundred full-time employees.

Congratulations, you improved a little over last year. Maybe you're below average for your size company in your industry, etc. But excuse me for asking:

How does knowing those stats actually help you make people safer?

For starters, specifically what twelve injuries occurred each month for the last two years? Let's say you actually separated out hand injuries from say, eye, foot, and back injuries. Now, what specific machine? At the end of the shift or the beginning of the shift? Were the workers wearing their gloves? Were they new or experienced workers? Trained or untrained? What kind of gloves, specifically, were they wearing at the time?

Those kinds of details might actually help you *do* something to prevent future injuries. Might actually allow you to *take action*. Truth is, unless you have really a lot of detail on injuries, there's no way for you to look for patterns and see how to change those patterns. No way for you to realize that, "Hey, those old drill presses really create a huge damn problem."

LAGGING VS. LEADING INDICATORS

Here's another statistic that might help you actually improve safety in the future:

How many average training hours did new hires complete this year, compared to last?

In chapter nine, we'll be doing a deep dive on gathering stats, but I want to offer this important preview: The number of injuries you've had on a monthly basis is what's known as a *lagging indicator*. The number of training hours you performed is what's known as a *leading indicator*.

Leading indicators show what positive steps are being taken to reduce injuries, and attempt to see if a company is working on reducing its injury rates. Specific leading indicators are critical stats for you, as a safety manager, to develop and track.

Other leading indicators for hand safety:

- What projects were undertaken to increase safety infrastructure? How many were completed or are underway?
- What research is being done on proper gloves? How many glove/job pairings were improved?
- What efforts are underway to find better trainers? How are those trainers performing? Are there any measurable results from the training in its present form?
- How many translations of safety signs into multiple languages were completed this year? How many remain?

WHO SEES YOUR STATS, AND WHO USES THEM?

A big problem with all statistics is who gets to see them. Companies have an incentive first to keep only very general statistics, like number of injuries per year; and second to show them to a very limited number of people.

Both of those incentives work against safety.

People on the floor or out on a rig need very specific stats to help them find and reduce dangers. People at the executive level need to be open about what's happening and what's being done to fix it. People have to talk, and they need hard data when they talk.

Indeed, the more people at the top know what's going on, the more likely they are to become involved, to care, to allocate necessary monies, and to take safety goals *personally.*

That makes keeping genuine, meaningful stats a vital part of any safety manager's job. You must see stats as a critical tool for moving the company forward. You must never see them as just a blank to fill in on a government form or a box to check on a corporate bylaw.

THE ELEPHANT IN THE ROOM

I was tempted to add one more common mistake to this list, but the subject was too big to boil down to a few paragraphs.

You might even say it's the elephant in the room.

Let's call it, "Failing to understand the psychology of hand injuries, both at the worker and the management level."

That elephant requires a whole chapter. And it comes next.

CHAPTER THREE

THE PSYCHOLOGY OF HAND SAFETY

If you want to keep people's hands safe, you have to start by understanding their brains.

The human brain includes a marvelous but imperfect warning system. This warning system picks up on a startling array of dangers in its surroundings—but it can easily be misled and distracted. Its observations can be dead wrong. Its fantastic radar can be put to sleep.

In this chapter, we'll start by looking at *cognitive biases*, a fancy term for the ways a brain gets tricked. Then we'll look at *mindfulness*, which is nothing but a New Age way of saying "staying alert."

From there, we'll move from the individual brain to *group think:* How do those around us influence our safety and our biases? How does their sex, their age, their culture of origin affect their safety? What about the psychology and mindset of the organization in which they work?

Eventually, we'll get to the proper and improper uses of *fear*.

A WORD ABOUT BBS

For those in the know, I'm sure a red flag went up when you read the title of this chapter and those first few paragraphs, and that flag was imprinted with the acronym "BBS." "Ah," you thought, "this chapter is about behavior-based safety, and I know that's trouble."

BBS is a strategy that approaches safety primarily from the standpoint of the worker's mindset, as part of the company's overall job in providing safe equipment and practices. Sometimes that strategy has been used to wrongly assign blame to "dumb worker behaviors" in an accident, instead of to "company policies, infrastructure, and processes."

So yes, there's a danger in over-focusing on the psychology of the worker, instead of the responsibility of the company.

On the other hand, BBS training has sometimes greatly helped workers improve their personal caution, mindfulness, and regard for one another's safety. We'll talk more about BBS at the end of this chapter. At this point, let me just say that in this book, we are here to learn from everyone: those who love BBS and those who hate it with a passion. Like everything, BBS has its uses and its abuses, and we're going to deal with both as we go along.

And just to be clear...this chapter is not about BBS. It's about the brain.

LIZARD BRAIN AND ANALYTIC BRAIN

Along with the individual mind and the group mind, there's another way of dividing up the way our brains function: lizard brain and analytic brain. Both assess risk and make decisions. Both are needed to function safely in the world. Both can be tricked.

Our lizard brain is the automatic, instinctive part of our mind that's always scanning the environment, looking for lions that might be hiding behind trees. Or rocks that might fall. Or open blades that might cut our fingers. It decides and moves instantly, *without thinking,* as long as it is awake.

Our analytic mind moves much more slowly. It sits and thinks. It makes lists of potential hazards and ranks them in priority. It considers pros and cons, reviews previous data points, and importantly, it *requires conscious effort to use.*

The two halves of our brain often function at the same time and ignore one another. When you're driving, you may be thinking about a problem at work and entirely forget that you are driving. All of a sudden you're home, and you think, "How did I get here?" Well, your lizard brain got you there while your analytic mind was doing its own thing.

Not only are both halves crucial to safety, but both can be fooled pretty much in equal measure. The lizard brain can ignore that smaller tree behind which a lion really is about to pounce. The analytic brain can forget to include trees on its list of hazards at all.

Which brings us to cognitive biases.

WE'RE A HOT MESS OF COGNITIVE BIASES

When we humans make decisions with our lizard or our analytic brains, we follow all kinds of assumptions based on what has happened to us before, what others have told us, and what we see right in front of our eyes. Without these *natural biases* we wouldn't really be able to function, as we wouldn't be able to make any decisions at all.

When these biases mislead us, it's not so much that they're flaws in the way we think, it's more that the pathways we *normally and habitually* take in making decisions, whether fast or slow, have created dangers.

A lot of safety depends on changing the normal and habitual way we see dangers and make decisions, so we will make safer decisions. To do that, we first have to be consciously aware of our biases.

And yes, this applies to both management and workers.

In this slim book, we can only hit the highlights of cognitive bias. Encyclopedias can be and have been written on the subject.[30]

OVERCONFIDENCE BIAS

Duh, right? Hardly anyone considers themselves overconfident, but nearly everyone is. Again, like all biases, we might not really be able to function in the world without at least a little overconfidence. From a safety perspective, however, it's close to the top of dangerous biases. Put simply:

> Most people believe they are more agile and smarter, as well as better at most tasks, than they actually are.

To go back to the driving example, do you believe that you are an above-average or below- average driver? No less than 93 percent of people who respond to that question say they are above average—and surely half of them are wrong.[31] This would not be a problem, unless you think that being above average gives you the ability to text and drive safely. Or weave through traffic.

The Hidden Dangers of Overconfidence

But it gets more subtle than that.

Overconfidence also leads us to trust ourselves to do a task at all times equally well, when our performance actually varies greatly.

In driving, we don't account for night, or a drink, or emotional upset, or momentary loss of attention.

In the workplace, overconfidence translates to doing things like skipping safety processes, assuming we can work as safely at 4 p.m. as we did at 10 a.m., ignoring the fact that the floor is understaffed that day, not getting help when we need it, assuming we know how a machine functions under all conditions—the list goes on and on.

In short, overconfidence leads us to skip best practices we know we should do.

We all know the moment when we think, "I have this skill, I've honed it, I don't need to follow the rules anymore. The rules are for people who don't know what they're doing." Or simply, "I can do this quicker if I leave out step three."

The worst thing about overconfidence is that you get positive reinforcement all the way up until disaster strikes.

Yes, you really can use that table saw without the guard, and the work really does go faster, and you've been doing it that way for years without any problem until, well, until you lose a finger. If you're doing something in an unsafe way, and you do it 500 times without injury, you start forgetting that it's unsafe. Then you get to 501.

Who's fooled by overconfidence? Both our lizard brain and our analytic brain. Lizard brain no longer sees the danger. Analytic brain has *quite consciously* dropped the risk from its hazard assessment list.

Go and watch an experienced worker who has been doing a dangerous job injury-free for twenty years. What have they been doing wrong for those twenty years that may break a finger tomorrow?

IGNORING BLIND SPOTS

Humans rarely walk into a room and ask, "What is it I don't see here?"

Lizard brain is especially bad at this, because it takes *conscious effort* to look for things that are not immediately obvious—just as it takes conscious effort to look into your blind spots when you make a lane change while driving. Such a search requires use of your analytic mind, which may or may not be doing its job to support its lizard partner.

A worker uses a knife to trim the excess off an extruded plastic part. Her attention is on her knife, on the part she is holding, on the speed of the line. Without looking, she puts her hand down to grab a clamp—unaware that another worker has left an open knife on the table. When she cuts herself, she is the victim of a cognitive bias in her lizard brain that assumes nothing has changed in the environment to endanger her.

Never before has a worker left a knife there—so her habituation to the environment has caused a blind spot. Part of this bias comes from the efficient and automatic tracking of the lizard brain. The lizard brain doesn't step back and wonder, "Hey, could a knife be left behind by that worker?" It just reaches out, as fast as it can, to grab the clamp.

The Danger in Obvious Dangers

Sometimes obvious dangers can cause blind spots to less obvious dangers.

Suppose, for example, a factory has a metal-stamping machine which has crushed workers' hands several times in the past, causing horrible injuries. When working with this machine, everyone watches the stamper like a hawk. Meanwhile, there's also an automatic arm that moves each piece of metal out of the way for the next to be stamped. It has exposed gears that can pinch and destroy a finger, but no one has ever experienced that injury. This automatic arm may be a blind spot danger—unseen, though even closer to a hand. *Hidden by the obvious danger.*

In the same analytic way that drivers can be trained to look in their blind spots, so can workers—and, perhaps more importantly, so can managers. Indeed, it's part of every manager's job to proactively look for and mitigate the unseen dangers their workers might encounter. This is especially true when there has been any change to an environment which the workers might not notice or account for. You might even say that the manager's job is to wake up the analytic brain that the worker may have let sleep as they became accustomed to their work.

What happened when you moved that machine? Did it put the workers dangerously close to another part of the line?

CONFIRMATION BIAS

The confirmation bias refers to the natural human tendency to "search for, interpret, favor, and recall information in a way that confirms our pre-existing beliefs or hypotheses."[32]

In other words, we often see only what we expect to see.

Safety expert, Thomas Krause, relates an incident in which a miner with thirty years' experience died when the roof of a tunnel collapsed.[33] The collapse came right after he and an equally experienced foreman had inspected the tunnel for structural issues, and found none. After the incident, an investigation found no less than 137 missing bolts, along with obviously compromised roof planks.

How had the foreman and the miner not seen these problems? The answer was simple: they'd done previous inspections of other tunnels in this mine without seeing any problems, so they didn't expect to see any in this tunnel.

Not only do we see what we expect to see, but our pre-programmed brains actively ignore anything that contradicts our first assumptions. This is true when we listen for news that confirms our political beliefs, and it's true when we work with our hands.

If we're used to seeing a drill lock lever in place, we may literally not see that the lock is up.

If we're used to turning off a machine when we go to lunch, we may literally not notice that the machine is running when we come back from lunch.

If we've seen somebody changing the blade on a saw a hundred times, and every time, after they changed the blade, they reclosed the safety guard, we may literally not see that this time, the guard was left up. Even if the guard is bright orange and at an obviously wrong angle.

If you hire a worker with a great resume of long experience, you expect to hear certain answers to your safety questions in an interview. When you actually ask the questions, you will tend to interpret his answers the way you want to hear them, ignoring clues that he doesn't actually know what he's doing.

The best antidote to the confirmation bias is the checkoff list. Pilots are forced to go through pre-flight checkoffs, and recent efforts to force surgeons to do pre-surgery checkoffs have shown huge reductions in surgical errors.[34]

Of course, checkoff lists are only as good as the person doing the checking off. Only as reliable as their diligence and their awareness of their own confirmation biases.

Where in your workplace could you use a checkoff to ensure hand safety? Who would you trust to do the inspection? Will they take the confirmation bias problem seriously?

See also chapter seven for a broader discussion of hazard assessments.

IGNORING THE BASELINE

All of us tend to think that our own circumstances are somehow unique, and we tend to ignore the typical statistics governing our activities. That includes accident rates.

This cognitive bias has a name: "ignoring the baseline."

For example, parents tend to dote on their own children, and often assume they will be good drivers when they turn sixteen—with an accident rate different than all the other sixteen-year-olds who came before. Insurance companies know better.

Smokers often assume that lung cancer just won't happen to them, even though statistics show otherwise. Once again, insurance companies know better.

We all know that overeating causes numerous medical conditions, but somehow we assume that we, ourselves, are immune from those conditions. Even overweight doctors seem to have this cognitive bias.

More than ignoring the baseline, we are often in active denial about the baseline.

A company may be using vibrating equipment like pneumatic drills. Over time, equipment like this can cause the serious condition called hand-arm vibration syndrome (HAVS) which we described in chapter one. Fingers become white, desensitized, and worse. Unless a company does the research on the baseline consequences of this kind of work, they will be completely unaware that this condition can (and will) occur over time. Just as likely, they already know about HAVS, but somehow just assume it's not going to happen to their people.

Even though workers have heard about their fellows developing serious conditions from, say, handling fiberglass insulation without gloves, they continue to do it—assuming, somehow, that it won't happen to them.

Maybe ignoring the baseline is a case of our lizard brains repressing our analytic brains and saying, "just get it done!" without thinking about the consequences. If so, the analytic brain must be taught to fight back.

As a safety manager, that means deeply understanding the typical risks faced by workers in your industry. It means doing the homework and overcoming this bias in your company culture.

If you're in the food processing industry, your workers are likely to face carpal tunnel syndrome. If you're running a small construction unit, your workers face a higher risk than workers on larger projects, with more safety inspections and controls in place—it's just true.[35]

How do you convince both supervisors and workers to consider the baseline? How do you convince them that they are not, in fact, safer than everyone else who ever did this job?

DEFAULT BIAS

Whenever a choice is presented to us, we tend to choose the defaults—it's not just easier and quicker, but we assume that the defaults are somehow the safest bet.

That means that when a worker approaches a task or a machine, they always tend to look for the defaults—whether someone else has explained the other options, or not.

This powerful bias makes the choosing and communicating of defaults a major responsibility of management.

If you have five different kinds of gloves available in the workplace, you need to make it absolutely clear which are the default gloves for a particular kind of work, or the work in general. That might mean a big picture of the default gloves next to a particular machine, or better yet a rack with those specific gloves placed next to the machine.

It also means that the defaults for that machine—safety guards, speed settings, etc.—need to be absolutely clear, both in training and in daily setup. The communication of defaults can be subtle.

A supervisor can say, "Mix these two chemicals together. Here's a bucket of gloves you can use to protect your hands." Or a supervisor can say, "Put on these gloves, then mix these two chemicals together." Only in the second way did the supervisor clearly communicate the gloves as a default, rather than a choice, thus greatly reducing the risk to workers.

Another phrase for "defaults" is "standard operating procedure." An SOP should not be violated without good reason.

You cannot expect workers to analyze each situation and make choices which are not presented as defaults. Their lizard brain will override their analytic brain every time and dive in with whatever they perceive as the default situation. This is not "stupidity," it's just the natural way everyone's brain operates.

If you have never done this, do it now.

Ask what are the defaults for each task from each worker? Have they been properly and fully defined? Are they the safest alternatives? How does the worker know, instantly, what the default choice should be? How is the default presented?

The Danger in Defaults

Sometimes, however, the default bias presents a real and present danger.

For example, a risk assessment may have a bunch of default checkoffs that people don't actually read through, but just choose the default options. It makes a big difference on a form whether you arrange all the "yes" bubbles on one side and all the "no" bubbles on the other, or mix them up so people don't just check off down one side or the other, by default.

Even worse is a pre-filled risk assessment, photocopied to save time.

The same thing can happen with safety meetings, in which the default is for no one to complain or raise an issue. Everyone "just knows" these meetings are intended to be short and uneventful, just to fulfill a bureaucratic requirement. The default is "routine and meaningless."

Has your company introduced a default safety checkoff of one kind or another which is creating danger?

UNDERESTIMATING CUMULATIVE RISK

Humans tend to vastly underestimate cumulative risk—the things that are harming them slowly, over time.

Everyone knows about frogs and boiling water. If you drop a frog into a pot of boiling water, it will jump out safely. But if you put the foolish amphibian in cold water and boil it slowly, it will not recognize the danger in time, and it will die. Unfortunately, this analogy can be applied again and again to hand safety.

People handle "just a little bit" of a dangerous chemical every day until they develop skin conditions or neurological issues or cancer.

People use vibration tools which are causing neurological damage over several years without noticing until it's too late.

Gloves wear thin and get holes, but people keep on using them. If these gloves had been issued on day one, they would never have been accepted.

The cutting room was safe when two people were working side by side. But then there's three. Then five. Then ten.

The line wasn't too dangerous when the stamper was set to five hits per minute, but now it's set to seven per minute.

The gears worked every time when the machine was new, but now the guys are recklessly smacking the gears with the palms of their hands to get the mechanism moving.

A Series of Small Compromises

A perhaps more insidious form of cumulative bias arises from the multiplication of small risks which creates a large risk. For example, in the Deepwater Horizon oil rig accident of 2010 in which eleven people died and seventeen were injured, safety investigators found no one single cause. Rather, it was a series of relatively minor safety compromises, made over a period of time, which together brought catastrophe.

Experience had taught the leaders and supervisors of the rig that their "small compromises" made to keep on schedule, were unlikely to be detected, and even less likely to cause a blowout. They never saw the cumulative risk they were creating.[36]

The Myth of the Safety Pyramid

Partly, the Deepwater Horizon risk was created by the mistaken thinking of the "safety pyramid." The myth of the safety pyramid insidiously combines a blindness to cumulative risk with a fallacious kind of statistical overconfidence.

Transocean, which operated the rig, had an excellent safety record—which meant that they recorded a very low number of minor accidents and near misses. Hence they thought they had a low risk of a major disaster.[37] That's because the myth of the safety pyramid is that it takes a lot of minor accidents and near misses before you get a major accident like a fatality. Here's an actual example of a mistaken pyramid analysis from Conoco-Phillips:[38]

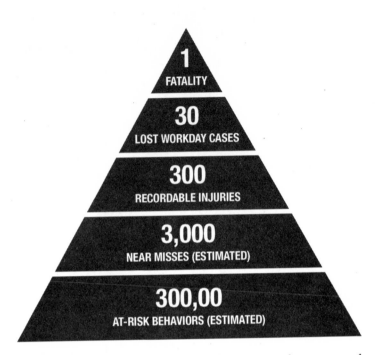

The idea is that you can predict the number of injuries and fatalities based on the numbers below in the pyramid: more minor stuff, more likely to have a major event.

When you step back and think about this pyramid logically, however, you can see its absurdity. *It only takes one at-risk behavior to create a fatality*, not 300,000. Also, you can be creating an enormous potential for a catastrophe without experiencing any minor disasters at all—which was the case on the Deepwater Horizon.

What cumulative risks are inevitable in your workplace? What cumulative risk does no one seem to notice?

RECENCY AND AVAILABILITY BIAS

The recency bias, also known as the "availability bias" of the human mind means that we tend to focus on top-of-mind, recent events, with lots of readily available information, giving them more importance than they deserve.

A good example might be airport security. Back in 2001 some guy tried to bomb a plane by hiding a device in his shoe—so immediately, airport security focused intensively on shoes, even though there were always plenty of other ways to hide bombs. In 2006 the same thing happened with small bottles of liquids. Now we all have to remove our shoes and dump our water bottles, even though the terrorists have moved on to testing new tricks.

The recency and availability bias means that we are always looking at the immediate past for answers, instead of looking forward.

The Danger of the "Accident Cycle"

If somebody loses a finger working with a harvester on a farm, everyone is going to be very careful around harvesters for a while. Attention will be paid to new gloves, guardrails, and protocols around harvesters. Meanwhile, workers are deploying pesticides bare-handed, they're fiddling with open tractor engines while the tractors are running, they're operating power takeoff flywheels without any training.

When we interviewed safety managers for this book, we heard plenty of complaints about upper management becoming obsessed with a recent accident, to the exclusion of long-term safety planning and training in other areas. "Somebody just lost a hand! I want you full time dealing with that. Never mind all that other safety BS you're working on!"

The lost hand was a tragedy, but the safety manager knew that it was an outlier injury, not a danger faced by many workers in every shift. Indeed, dangers may become *hidden* by the focus on this recent event, as no overall hazard assessments are taking place.

This tendency to focus on one event at a time creates what's known as "the accident cycle," in which management thinking focuses obsessively on one accident, brings that injury rate down, loses interest, and moves on to focus on the next accident—always thinking backward.

The accident cycle can even cause management to lose credibility with workers. As management begins issuing memos, speeches, and commands related to the last accident, workers may know of far more dangerous conditions which are not being addressed at all.

Are you prone to "accident cycle" thinking? How can you assure that your company makes consistent progress in all areas of safety, without becoming focused only on recent events?

THE PSYCHOLOGY OF PAYING ATTENTION

Nothing is more important to hand safety than paying attention, but nothing is more difficult to train for or control. Injuries often come from distraction, and distractions can come from anywhere.

Psychologists classify them as either external or internal, where they are named as either *sensory* or *emotional*.

Sensory distractions are, of course, many: from radios to cell phones to the new hunting cap the guy next to us decided to wear to work. Emotional distractions include the countless narratives always running through our heads: the fight we just had with a spouse, worries about job security, anger about a reprimand.

Some studies have shown that it's easier to distract modern people because we have become used to switching our attention faster and faster between screens, conversations, and the bright visual distractions in our environment. One study put some of us hard-to-focus modern people in a room with a computer and a TV, and found that we switched between the two on average every fourteen seconds. That's 120 times in 27.5 minutes.[39]

Modern workplaces, too, are rife with distractions, from computer monitors to signs to mobile phones.

But the problem of emotional distractions has probably always been as bad as it is today. Whenever people are doing a repetitive task they know well, they tend to put their lizard brains on autopilot to get the job done, while they let their analytic minds wander, process memories, think about the future: Where will I go for lunch? Is my wife still mad at me?

TRAINING LIZARD BRAIN

No matter how far our analytic brain wanders, our lizard brain tries its best to protect us. That's because lizard brain is doing more than its job on autopilot, it's waiting for *triggers* to instantly change its focus and bring analytic brain back into the room.

When our forebears were tilling soil or gathering berries or grinding acorns, part of their lizard brains were always monitoring their environment for danger. Or, to be more precise, their lizard brains were keyed to certain sights and sounds as triggers: birds startled from the brush, the sound of a snapping twig, a shadow behind a tree.

We can use our advanced analytic brain to program our own lizard brains to use certain triggers to bring us back to full consciousness and attention. We have all, for example, programmed our lizard brain to recognize the click of a seatbelt as a sound cue to focus on driving.

In the workplace, it's possible to train yourself to other triggers. You can train your lizard brain that when you put on your gloves, your mind needs to go into full work focus. When you flip that switch on a machine. When you hear the conveyor belt start.

We can be aided by our use of simple triggers like caffeine—morning coffee being the most common cue that it's time to get serious and pay attention.

Some people are better at this kind of *cognitive control* than others, but cognitive control can be trained in anyone. For example, people have designed computer-based training applications that use game-like stimuli to do this training.[40]

LIZARD BRAIN NEEDS BREAKS

The most common way to reset attention and get people to focus on a task is also probably the best: the break.

Even a short intermission can act as a refresh button on attention, not just because lizard brain gets tired, but because the "return to work" trigger puts lizard brain back on alert to be careful and do the job properly.

One study gave participants a fifty-minute task requiring close attention on a computer. Half were given no breaks during the fifty minutes, and half were given two, very short breaks. The people who got the two breaks did better in the fifty total minutes, both in amount of work accomplished, and the quality of the work.[41]

In other words, shorter bursts of high-quality focus can be safer and more productive than longer periods of lower-quality focus.

Short breaks are especially important when the work is repetitive or boring, because repetitive work can put both lizard brain and analytic brain to sleep, creating dangerous inattention through a kind of hypnosis. Everyone, for example, is familiar with the dangers of "highway hypnosis" on a long drive—the only cure being short breaks to bring the mind back on track.

MINDFULNESS

The New Age term for paying attention is *mindfulness.*

Why would a new term be needed? Because mindfulness is a much broader concept. To be safe, you need to do *more than pay attention to the task at hand, you need to be mindful of the overall situation around you.* You need to be mindful of your own state of health, the time of day, and the safety cues in your immediate environment.

Mindfulness implies that a worker is trying to stay *in the present tense.* Soldiers, emergency responders, and others who must make split-second decisions call it *situational awareness.*

Whatever you call it, it means the mind is not reliving the past or anticipating the future. It means the mind is undistracted by emotional narratives, and actively shutting out sensory distractions. It's right "here."

What are other people doing in your immediate area? What is the state of cleanliness of the work space? Analytic brain asks: What hidden danger is represented by the fact that you *did* have an argument with your spouse, that you *are* worried about your job security? Do you need to slow down your work because your focus is waning as it gets closer to lunch hour (studies have shown that in some settings, hand injuries spike between 10-11 a.m.)[42] or because you are on the night shift?[43]

Can mindfulness be taught?

Training programs have indeed been created that use meditation to train the mind to focus, but partly mindfulness is simply *an attitude* that can be encouraged or discouraged by both supervisors and peers.

If a supervisor just says, "Okay, take a ten-minute break," it's very different than saying, "Okay, take a ten-minute break. This is dangerous stuff and you need to come back fresh and focused."

In the second case, the supervisor is treating workers like adults, not children. He or she admits the work is dangerous, presents the problem, and urges workers to find a personal solution and work on their mindfulness.

It's not that workers are children who need a recess, it's that they are adults who must use their break to produce the mindfulness that will protect them in dangerous work—and keep them productive, too.

Better yet, the supervisor could say, "It's late in the day, and everyone's tired. Tired makes for accidents, people. I don't want you to get hurt, and you don't want you to get hurt. Let's take a break, and then we'll all focus and do this last hour of the day safely."

ANALYTIC BRAIN MUST DIRECT AND TRAIN LIZARD BRAIN

In the case above, the supervisor is telling workers to use their analytic brain to rest and train their lizard brain.

Lizard brain does not operate independently of analytic brain. Indeed, lizard brain knows that analytic brain is the boss, and it will take direction and training from its boss. Analytic brain must seize this power and embrace this responsibility. It must also remember that lizard brain needs constant reminders and constant repetition to develop things like "muscle memory."

Analytic brain must also take the time, again and again, to make lizard brain aware of the cognitive biases we discussed earlier.

Analytic brain must tell lizard brain to stop and become aware of the environment: who else is working, what machines are moving, how worn out the gloves may be.

Analytic brain must actively find triggers for the high alert and focus of lizard brain.

PREPARING THE MIND

Analytic brain can also participate with lizard brain in imagining doing a task safely before actually doing the task. All athletes do this, and as I mentioned, everyone who works with their hands is a kind of athlete. Just as an athlete pictures vaulting over a pole before actually running down the track and doing the vault, so can a worker on an oil rig imagine the steps in changing out a drill bit safely before actually doing it.

How can workers be taught to prepare their minds for safe work? Would your workers even be open to a "touchy feely" program like this? Here's a suggestion which you can modify for your particular circumstances. Maybe you'll find a way to make it acceptable to your people—at least some part of it. Every group is different.

1. Before beginning their shift, ask workers to take a calming breath and try to relax their minds from worry and distractions—bringing themselves into the present moment. Ask them to close their eyes and focus for a moment simply on their breathing.

2. Beyond their breathing, workers can then expand their attention to become aware of their environment: the traffic zooming by their worksite, the forklifts in motion, the other workers, the way the tools are laid out, the way their gloves feel, the time of day.

3. Next, ask workers to imagine doing their task in the best and safest manner, actually running through all the steps ahead of time in their minds. Tell them that athletes like tennis players and pole vaulters and swimmers do this every single time, before they compete. Tell the workers they are athletes too. As they do this, their analytic minds will run through the dangers, automatically—not in fear, but in a calm, controlled way.

4. Then, if possible, have workers physically do the safe motions, over and over, to develop "muscle memory."

5. All along, tell them that the goal is to maintain a clear mind which is calm and aware and not lulled into dangerous inattention. It can help to go back to bringing the attention to the breath throughout the workday. This centers the mind, clears it, and makes it aware and open.

6. Now, ask workers to schedule for themselves tiny mental breaks, perhaps less than fifteen seconds every now and then, in which they repeat steps one through three, very briefly, for a mental reset before continuing work. This is especially important before beginning a new task, but workers should monitor their own attention from time to time and pull back for a "performance break." "Am I paying attention? Am I rushing this? Do I have all the tools and protective gear I need? Is someone near me putting me in danger?"

7. A bit more advanced: Ask workers to consider creating a little trigger that reminds them to act in a safe manner. Their trigger might be putting on their gloves, going back to the active face of the mining pit, turning on their equipment, calling out "ready" to a coworker. *Any trigger will do, but lizard brain wants and expects a trigger to bring it into focus.*

This kind of training might be more acceptable to your workers if it takes place in a training environment like a classroom, but it will be most effective at the worksite. Maybe a prep in the classroom, then repeated at the worksite? Try it.

With true mindfulness, analytic brain is *always* doing this active kind of management for lizard brain. With true mindfulness, analytic brain is always keeping lizard brain on track.[44]

THE CHALLENGE OF MINDFULNESS TRAINING

As I read over the suggested mindfulness exercises above, I realize how important it is to adapt them to the reality of a particular workplace. One size does not fit all.

Marissa Afton consults in industrial safety with the Potential Project, and sometimes does mindfulness training. She's very aware of the challenge in trying to do mindfulness training for industrial workers: "Just telling people that their brains will, naturally, go on autopilot when they're doing repetitive tasks doesn't necessarily help them—it just helps them know that they are sometimes at risk without [deciding] to be at risk. It's not the knowledge that's getting in the way, it's the lack of tools."[45]

Providing people with those tools, however, is a challenge. For starters, she doesn't necessarily like to use the word "mindfulness," and instead tries to talk about "situational awareness" or use other words that resonate with workers. Basically, "how are we continually sharpening our focus and opening our awareness to both seen and unseen risks? How do we go to the mental gym? People who work in corporate environments take well to the idea of sitting and breathing as a mind-training practice. It fits into the natural workday. *But for people always on the move, just sitting still can be really uncomfortable—physically uncomfortable. I ask them, 'What does it mean to move with sharp focus and also a sense of relaxation?'"*

A good trainer can use the feedback from such a conversation to re-purpose the suggested training program for an environment where it would make no sense to sit and meditate.

See Appendix 4 for some mindfulness resources.

THE ROLE OF FEAR

You may be surprised that so far in this chapter, I've not talked a lot about fear. After all, what focuses the mind better than fear? What inspires safe behavior more than knowing that a wrong move can remove a finger?

Safety experts know, however, that fear is a double-edged sword. Fear can motivate or distract. Fear can focus the mind or throw it into denial. Fear can cause the mind to go into a deliberate, analytic approach or it can produce "deer in the headlights" paralysis. Use fear in the wrong way, and it can definitely backfire.[46]

The surest way to produce fear for their hands is to show workers pictures of horribly mangled hands. Pictures really are worth a thousand words. In this way, the psychologist might assert, a worker can experience the consequences of an accident without having to go through an accident—thereby changing behavior.

But *should* you show people pictures of horribly mangled hands? Should you also show them videos of realistically designed dummy hands being shredded by a table saw?[47] The answer is a hearty *maybe*. These pictures and videos are readily available, and studies have sometimes validated their use—but the precise circumstances have always mattered, a lot.

Let's make some rules, based on long experience at leading companies, on the use of fear:

1. Never forget that the use of images is far different than the use of words. Fear is generally a visceral response to a visual image, if only an image in the mind.
2. Never show a picture of a horribly mangled hand without

it being specifically relevant to the machinery or tasks of the audience. Generic pictures are a bad idea, as they create free-floating anxiety, with no solution.

3. Never show a mangled hand without immediately offering the safe, secure alternative practice to prevent it. The worker needs to believe that the proposed behavior is actually effective and that they have the ability to do it. Otherwise, the mind will go into denial, and the topic will be avoided altogether.

4. Never show the result of a very recent injury, in which the audience might know the person, relatives of the person, or friends of the person involved. This will be seen, rightly, as a terrible violation of personal privacy. If someone in the audience saw the accident, it may also trigger a kind of PTSD.

5. Never post a graphic photo of an injury next to the machine at which it occurred. This will cause nonstop anxiety which will not lead to safety, but to mental blocks. Indeed, people will block out that image in order to do the work, and it will become counterproductive over time. You can use such an image in training (see below), but not permanently on display. This is especially bad if you forget rule three above, and don't show the right way to do the job safely.

But Sometimes Only Graphic Images Create **Believability**

All that said, fear, even horror, can and should be a vital part of creating *believability for warnings*. So, even after all those rules, I'm not telling you to banish horrible pictures from your training sessions.

Believability is vital, because humans have a natural tendency to think that bad things will not happen to them personally. Seeing a picture of a mangled hand associated with a particular task can make a worker finally believe that it's possible, there's a real threat, and might happen to them.

Driver-training programs use horrible images of accidents to make drivers safer. In some countries, putting pictures of horrible cancers right on cigarette packages reduces the likelihood of people buying cigarettes.[48]

In an industrial setting, believability is especially important for long-term, cumulative injuries, like the HAVS vibration syndrome, chemical exposures, and the like.

So, here are some more rules about using fear:

1. As part of creating believability, it's important that your graphic examples be drawn from ethnic, cultural, and gender groups similar to your workers. Because of the powerful denial factor in the human psyche, if you only see that someone from another race or culture was injured, you are that much less likely to believe that it could be you.
2. Your horror stories must include the long-term consequences of an injury. This includes repeated surgeries, lost hand mobility, family consequences, and the like. Part of combatting fatalism is to combat the idea that an injury is a one-off terrible event that happens, and then it's over. Take a look again at those training exercises with the taped up fingers, simulating lost digits, that we discussed back in chapter one.
3. It's important to rotate out horrible images used in training. Seeing the same image over and over will cause people to block it out and ignore it.

But once again, read the "never" rules carefully. Graphic photos on cigarette cartons work partly because people don't have to smoke. Actually posting photos next to machines people have to use will cause a very different, and bad reaction, than using the photos briefly in training sessions.

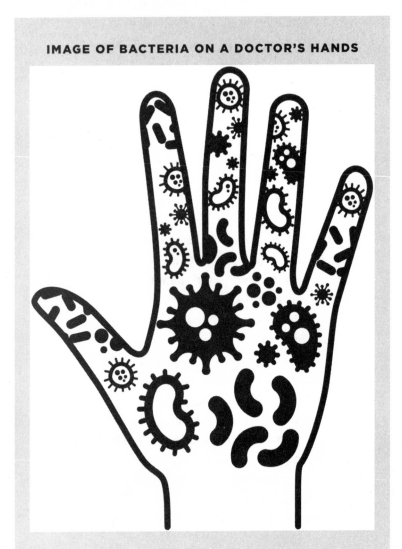

IMAGE OF BACTERIA ON A DOCTOR'S HANDS

The Freakonomics authors, Stephen Dubner and Steven Levitt,

document a case study on the use of graphic images at Cedars Sinai Hospital in the early 2000s. The hospital decided they needed to get their handwashing rate up among doctors. When everything from incentives to penalties made no difference, an administrator tried a different tactic.

At a weekly meeting of the supervising physicians, the administrator had each doctor press their palms into a Petri dish, and sent the dishes to the lab to be cultured. The spreading colonies of bacteria in the shape of the doctors' hands were photographed and doctors were sent their photos. One especially bad and disgusting example of an anonymous doctor "Bob" was briefly turned into a screensaver throughout the hospital's computers.

Handwashing shot up to around 100 percent and the good results continued long after the experiment was over.[49]

Why did this work? The doctors finally believed the problem was real, and concerned their own hands. Graphic, even disgusting evidence is sometimes needed to create believability, hence safety. But this tactic must be used carefully and wisely.

THE PSYCHOLOGY OF CULTURAL NORMS

The culture in which a worker was raised plays a huge role in their personal safety psychology. It directly affects how they act in risky situations and how they relate to management as it tries to enforce safety protocols.

Age also plays a role. Generational differences play a role. Gender plays a role. And yes, how these factors *interact* matters in the moment a worker reaches for a tool.

I'm not going to get into specific cultural norms here, by country and geography—because it's stupid to make generalizations about specific cultures without adding in a hundred if, ands, and buts. One truth may apply generally to a national character, and one truth may apply only to the countryside, or the big city, or may be misguided, or may have gone completely out of date.

But it's equally stupid to say such differences do not exist or should be ignored.

As a manager you have a vital responsibility to get as far inside workers' heads as you can. That means getting an understanding of their cultural norms, and really understanding how they differ from the norms you grew up with.

There are cultures where people speak up when they see something going awry, and cultures in which they keep quiet—even when lives are at stake.

Cultures in which people report accidents, and cultures in which accidents are ignored and covered up.

Cultures in which fatalism (accidents are inevitable and foreordained) plays a critical role, and cultures in which fatalism is considered primitive and absurd (nothing is foreordained).

Cultures in which rules are followed by default, and cultures where rules are broken by default.

Cultures in which people assume their hands will get beat up or fingers lost in the course of their working lives, and cultures in which one bad cut is considered a tragedy.

Cultures where people look you in the eye when they're paying attention, and cultures in which they feign indifference while actually listening closely.

Cultures where the men take chances, scoff at wearing gloves, and joke about safety to show "machismo."

Cultures where the women in traditional male occupations take additional risks to show they are as tough as the guys.

Cultures where people will publicly disagree with you, and cultures where no one ever disagrees with anyone in front of a group, especially an authority figure.

You see where I'm going. When you stand up and give a safety talk to a bunch of folks about to head into a dangerous situation, and you want them to actually be safe, you'd better know who the heck you are talking to.

In fact, even if you hail from the same national culture as your workers, I'll bet you haven't taken enough time to step back and examine the cultural norms that are endangering your people. Indeed, most of us get so used to these norms, that we stop seeing them.

FATALISM IN CANE CRUSHERS

A 2001 study[50] of sugar cane crushers in India revealed some startling cultural norms. Injury rates were astronomical in this work because the crushing machines, used to extract juice, had exposed rollers with highly inadequate safety guards, and none of the workers studied used gloves—partly due to the cost, as individuals would have to supply their own gloves. However, when questioned outside of the workplace, only 16 percent of workers felt that machines with improved safety features were required, and only 40 percent thought special gloves would help, with 19 percent saying gloves would be an actual hindrance. More than half the workers put in over twelve hours a day, but 88 percent did not consider "long duration of work" a hindrance or a danger. Some 63 percent thought that injuries came from "carelessness," 50 percent thought that injuries were due to "bad luck," and 38 percent attributed the injuries to "God's will."

What happens when a person with this background moves to a country with higher standards and expectations for safety? How can their attitude be changed?

THE ROLE OF AGE

You will not be surprised to learn that according to academic studies, risk-taking behavior does generally decrease with age.[51] Maybe it's something in our genes or hormones, or maybe it's just that older people have seen that bad things do, indeed, happen. Even to them. As you would assume, younger workers do have higher accident rates in industrial settings. Not just through lack of experience, but through lack of carefulness.[52]

Generationally, however, the data is sometimes reversed, at least for certain factors. In our present time, for example, so-called millennials may be more likely to wear gloves for dangerous tasks than older baby boomers. Why? Because culturally, baby boomers often grew up in an environment where gloves weren't normally worn for similar tasks. Indeed, some experts say that decades from now, when millennials are in their fifties and sixties, they may act more safely than their present elders.

I've seen this myself. Plenty of times I've heard older workers say, "I don't need to wear any gloves" while a twenty-year-old will say, "Gloves are good. Gloves are normal. I'm fine with them." Sometimes it's more about a cultural time and place than age and hormones.

On the other hand, studies show that millennials dislike being observed and monitored, more than previous generations disliked it. They may also have thinner skins when it comes to criticism.[53]

Bottom line on age, generation, and culture? *Don't assume everyone thinks the way you do.* Indeed, we probably should have listed "assuming another person shares your safety values" under the cognitive biases section of this chapter. Or even in the top ten mistakes of chapter two.

The people you are trying to help may literally be willing to accept more risk than you would accept.

Your job is not to let them.

Never forget that rules and processes must override individual safety values, whether they arise from age, from generation, or from culture.

THE ROLE OF GENDER AND MARRIAGE

As you might expect, men get injured at a much higher rate on the job than women. But no one is quite sure whether that's because men engage in riskier behaviors than women, or because men are generally assigned to more dangerous tasks. Indeed, the difference narrows greatly when men and women are performing identical, or similar work.[54]

Anecdotally, most of us suspect that married people, especially with children, tend to work more safely and take fewer chances than singles. However, studies show that other factors may temper this effect.[55]

In short, it would be foolish for anyone to just assume that married people will act more responsibly, or that women will act more responsibly than men.

THE HASSLE FACTOR

An often-overlooked psychological factor in hand safety might be called the *hassle factor*. Question is, how much hassle will people tolerate in order to be safe? In this game, seconds matter. Even split seconds.

If a barrel full of gloves is located five feet away instead of twenty feet away from workers, it can mean low injury or high injury rates. If specialized gloves are hung on glove boards, with each hook clearly labeled for a task, it might mean that a worker spends five seconds less deciding which glove to use.

With this simple five-second reduction in hassle, the correct glove might be chosen 90 percent more often, and human hands might be saved.

If safety rails are up by default, instead of somebody having to spend five seconds raising the rail, fingers may be saved.

If you provide clips for workers to keep their gloves hanging from their belts when not being used, with the gloves ready and right at hand, you may increase glove use by a factor of ten.

One client saw that their workers were removing their metal-handling gloves to work a touch screen monitor. They asked my company to add touch screen compatibility to the gloves, and boom, glove use skyrocketed thanks to just this slight reduction in hassle.

Never forget that hassle matters. And a lot more than you think.

One of our clients realized his company was spending a lot on gloves, so he made a simple process change. Instead of putting out boxes of new gloves, ready for the taking, he made employees go ask their supervisors when they needed a new pair. As I discussed back in chapter two, this change also created an adverse psychological reaction—workers wondered, "Would the supervisors think they were stupid if they asked for new gloves? Dishonest?"

Hand injury rates shot up immediately. So did costs, thanks to increased medical expenses, lost time, and insurance rates. A year later, management gave up on the policy and started putting out big boxes of gloves again, all around the manufacturing floor.

Safety expert, Todd Grover, currently with Master Lock, has proposed the "15-second rule:" if you have to walk more than fifteen seconds to get the safety equipment you need, chances are you will think twice before using it to protect yourself.[56] The thought goes through your head, "Do I really need this?"

It's just human nature. You cannot fight it. So don't try. In fact, fifteen seconds may be too much.

Many companies have had success with "vending machines" for worker gloves. The machines are free, but workers have to punch in a unique code to get a new pair of expensive gloves. No personal interaction with a supervisor is needed, but the machines can be located close to the work, and there's at least some control and tracking over a valuable resource.

THE DISCOMFORT FACTOR

One of my safety consultants spent a day observing at a client's factory. Again and again, she saw one astonishing behavior: *Workers were taking off their gloves to perform their tasks, then putting the gloves back on afterwards.*

Why? Because the gloves were hot, sweaty, and too bulky for the task. Probably, the workers weren't even thinking about the absurdity of their action—it was just automatic, because the gloves were uncomfortable.

All safety experts struggle with the discomfort factor, not just in PPE, but in other safety infrastructures. Every safety manager must ask themselves—or actually, ask the workers—*beyond the hassle, how much discomfort will a person bear to be safe doing this job?*

Training matters in both discomfort and in hassle, of course. Psychologies can be shifted. Ultimately, however, it's the job of management to provide equipment people will actually use. That means gloves that aren't too bulky, aren't too hot for the climate, gloves that get replaced or laundered regularly so they don't smell, and of course, gloves that aren't provided just to cover the ass of management (see Mistake #8 in chapter two).

DO'S AND DON'TS OF FOCUSING ON WORKER BEHAVIOR

Way back at the beginning of the chapter I mentioned the inherent controversy in discussing BBS, or behavior-based safety. Sure enough, when I was researching this book, I ran into a lot of people who hated the whole idea of asking about the psychology of workers and how to make workers safer "in the moment." These people were pissed that I'd even posed the question.

You will find statements from unions, in particular, opposing the entire subject. As I mentioned, they worry because they have seen companies sometimes use BBS as a way to avoid responsibility for proper safety infrastructure, protective equipment, and policies. Instead of replacing worn-out equipment, for example, these companies would say, "It's the workers' fault. Let's focus on their behaviors because they aren't paying attention. It's not our problem, it's theirs."

My favorite image of BBS-hating comes from a United Steel Workers' presentation.[57] It shows a mouse wearing a crash helmet as it enters a mousetrap set with cheese. Obviously, the helmet ain't gonna help.

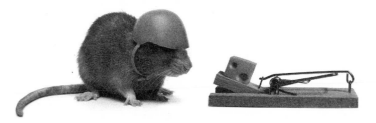

The union's point, again and again, is that the company should eliminate or reduce the hazard, rather than focusing on BBS, or even on personal protective equipment. They're right about that priority. Indeed, in chapter five, which discusses infrastructure, we will look closely at the "safety hierarchy" in which the number one goal of a company must be to eliminate a hazard, long before it goes down to the level of safety training, mindfulness, or PPE.

Fine.

But why not take all possible steps? Before BBS was conceived in the 1970s and 1980s, companies would focus *only* on processes, design, and PPE—psychology and worker behavior were entirely ignored. Management behavior was ignored as well. As I emphasized at the beginning of the chapter, if you read this book carefully, you will see that when I talk about behaviors, I'm not just talking about workers.

In fact, here's a kinder, gentler analogy than the mousetrap. You can think about modifications in worker behavior and psychology like vitamins. Vitamins can improve your health, but they aren't going to make up for a diet of burgers and fries. Your mom would say, "Get rid of the burgers and fries, and take your vitamins too."

The next chapter will be all about creating a culture of safety, starting in the boardroom. Without a culture of safety, the right infrastructure changes will not be made, the hazards will not be eliminated, the PPE will not be purchased, and no one will do the right training to keep worker behavior safe, either.

BBS GAMIFICATION

Here are two examples of implementing BBS in a friendly way with "gamification." That means creating a game to improve safe behaviors.

Hand injuries had been occurring with alarming frequency at an oil refinery—possibly due to the way workers were placing their hands on dangerous equipment and when performing dangerous work. In the first game, workers were asked to look at the way they and their coworkers placed their hands when performing a task. Everyone was given a set of green and yellow cards, and a bucket to throw them in.

Every time they saw an unsafe placement of hands, they were asked to throw a yellow card in the bucket. Every time they saw a safe placement, they tossed in a green card. A yellow might mean getting too close to a pinch point or carrying a load wrongly or without gloves. It had to be an action that actually put the person at risk of injury, such as slowly losing grip on a box and not setting it down to readjust the load. A green might mean wearing gloves or keeping fingers away from turning gears. It was simple, anonymous, nonjudgmental, and relied on the experienced eyes of the workers rather than the inexperienced eyes of management.

The game went on for three weeks, and over those three weeks the number of green cards steadily increased over the number of yellow. In the subsequent year, hand injuries were substantially reduced over the previous year.[58]

TAG—YOU'RE IT

Here's another game, based on the children's game of tag. On a construction site, workers were all given two pairs of gloves, one black-brown and one fluorescent orange. When one worker saw another putting their hands at risk, they were asked to point it out, and the other employee would have to switch to the bright orange gloves. Employees wearing orange gloves then became "it" and had to be on the lookout for others putting their hands at risk. They could only remove their own orange gloves when they spotted someone else and "tagged" them. Once again, the game showed dramatic improvements to hand safety.[59]

Importantly, however, games like this can only be attempted in a workplace where morale is high, management is trusted, and camaraderie already runs strong. I like to say that the devil of BBS is not so much in the details, but in the personalities. The right supervisor, standing up and introducing games like this to the right group in the right way, can make a huge difference in people's safety. The wrong supervisor, with the wrong attitude, trying this with the wrong worker culture could just annoy everyone.

DON'T MAKE COMMON MISTAKES IN A BBS PROCESS

There are dozens of books on BBS, and the full subject cannot be dealt with here. I highly recommend *The Behavior-Based Safety Process* by Thomas Krause,[60] a safety icon and pioneer in the field, as a starting point.

I will just say that if you head into a BBS process, you have to do it right, or you will indeed anger workers, and maybe even make workers less safe. Here are some rules when creating a behavior-based program, drawing from the original four-step process as outlined by Krause.

1. Identify hazards *and* behaviors, not just behaviors. When you do this identification, keep in mind all the cognitive biases we discussed earlier, especially the recency bias. Don't just focus on recent injuries or the obvious dangers. Involve workers and supervisors in the assessment. Use the hazard assessment processes we discuss in chapter seven. *Identify new hazards and you will earn trust.*

2. Gather data by observing the way work is done, but *also* by talking to the workers about what would make them safer. Don't hide your efforts, do them in public, in a cooperative way. *When people are asked for help, they are more likely to support you.*

3. Give feedback to workers *and* to management about what each could do to eliminate, reduce, or protect against the hazard. *This is important, but the very biggest mistake you can make is to stop at this step.* Lots of consulting companies out there will go through a BBS process and end with a study or a set of recommendations, with no follow-through by management.

4. It's not enough to give feedback, you have to make people safer. Indeed, failure to follow through will create a climate of distrust which will reduce, not improve safety. Indeed, when I spoke with Thomas Krause he complained bitterly that too many companies stopped their BBS process at "recommendations," giving BBS itself a bad name. So...

In step four, you have to take action. That action must ensure that the safety hierarchy outlined in chapter five is followed, which means that the company takes all possible steps in hazard reduction before addressing worker behavior. During this step, you also have to make sure that workers are involved in the actual changes and approaches of both infrastructure and behavior modification. When workers see action, their trust will be cemented.

5. Now I want to add a fifth step, which you will not necessarily find in the early literature on BBS, and that's "evaluate what happened." Did you indeed improve safety? Have the numbers actually improved? *Without such an analysis, you will not even know if step four occurred.* Speaking of stats, beyond looking back, you must also look at leading indicators which might predict reductions of injury into the future. For a full discussion on the use and abuse of stats like these, spend some quality time with chapter eight of this book.

These five rules apply not just to BBS, but to *every* recommendation in this book. If it's not a team effort with management and workers, it's not going to pay off for either. That *always* means an open, public effort to improve safety, not a consultant slinking around with a clipboard, observing workers and secretly recording unsafe behaviors, delivering a closed-door report to management.

BBS IN ACTION

Here's another example of an effective BBS initiative, done the right way.

A manufacturing company used long tables where workers

cut plastics, cardboard, and so forth with knives. They had a lot of hand injuries at these tables, so observers were sent to look at the work in action. They saw that many injuries resulted because knives were being left on the tables and grabbed or brushed accidentally. They discussed this with the workers, and came up with a mutual solution: create a series of sheaths attached to the edge of the table, where it would be handy to put the knives away.

But there was more. Volunteers from each shift agreed to stop their work for five minutes every day, take a clipboard, and make a note of how many knives were left out on the table. No names. No blame. Just numbers.

At the end of each week, they put up a chart that showed, "This is how many times knives were left on the table unsheathed this week." The first week it was around forty times. The second around twenty times. The numbers went way down from there—along with the injuries.

A study[61] at a major oil refinery showed that a behavior-based safety program reduced accidents by a staggering 81 percent. There were 79 percent fewer lost time cases and a 97 percent savings in worker compensation costs. Post-BBS implementation improved safety performance index scores by 29 percentage points. In this case, the study verified that actual injuries were reduced, not just the reporting of injuries (a vital step). Similar results have been seen in programs that followed the five-step BBS program outlined above, with all the caveats attached.

Similar studies have proven the effectiveness of BBS in many other contexts, with startlingly good results.[62]

THE CHAIN OF BEHAVIORS AND PSYCHOLOGIES

If you take away just one key message from this chapter on psychology and human behavior, take away this:

There is no such thing as individual behavior separate from group behavior. Changing individual behavior depends on changing group behavior, top to bottom. We live as fish in a school of fish, as birds in a flock of birds. We are members of a group psychology based on national culture, company culture, generational culture, etc., and etc., again.

Philosophers try to find the link between the *proximate* cause and the *distal* cause of an event—the near and distant cause. For safety managers, that means figuring out how the immediate, obvious cause of an accident is actually just the endpoint of a chain of events beginning with the not so obvious, ultimate cause which may be many bureaucratic layers and years separated from the event.

Here's an example of a proximate and distal chain of events leading to an accident. It's not a hand injury example, but I find it instructive.

NO ONE TO BLAME AND EVERYONE TO BLAME

On December 9, 2010, a dust explosion at a metal recycling facility in West Virginia killed three employees and seriously injured a fourth.[63]

The *proximate* cause of the explosion was determined quickly. A maintenance worker had installed an old, bad blade in a blending machine and returned it to service. Soon after, the bad blade began scraping the sides of the machine, causing sparks that caused a flash fire in the machine and then an explosion in the dust that hung in the air of the factory itself.

Installing a bad blade and restarting the machine was the last thing that anyone did to contribute to the incident, but it was hardly the whole story. First off, blades had been wearing out with increasing frequency in the big blender, and each time they were replaced, workers found more evidence that they were scraping the sides. New, somewhat better-fitting blades were sometimes available, and sometimes not; and these too were unreliable. Indeed, workers had previously put out small fires inside the blender. A large crack had recently been found in the wall of the blender, caused by the stress. It had been welded shut, and management had made the decision to continue work without having a reliable, overall solution to the problem.

On the day that the maintenance worker bent an old blade to make it fit, *he was actually doing the normal, expected thing*: making do in whatever way he could to keep work moving uninterrupted.

There were other distal causes of the disaster and deaths: Management knew about the problem of dust in the air, but had never addressed it properly. Evacuation plans were inadequate and not drilled. Material storage procedures were not followed, adding to the chaos. Emergency response was confused. And on and on.

It probably never occurred to the maintenance worker to think, "I shouldn't be doing this," and it certainly never occurred to him to say, "I'm calling for work to stop until this situation is fixed."

No one person was to blame, and everyone was to blame.

Which brings us to the next chapter, in which we try to figure out how to get everyone in a company to take responsibility, every single day.

CHAPTER FOUR

HOW TO TURN AROUND A COMPANY CULTURE

When all those people died on the Titanic on April 15, 1912 it wasn't the fault of the lookout who failed to spot the iceberg until about thirty-seven seconds before collision.

It wasn't the fault of the officer who failed to supply that lookout with binoculars because the cabinet was locked and no one had the key.[64]

It wasn't the fault of the captain who agreed to cross the ocean during iceberg season at high speed on his last voyage before retirement.

It wasn't the fault of company leaders who supplied only the legal minimum of lifeboats, far too few to accommodate all the passengers and crew.

It wasn't the fault of the engineers who designed the hull and watertight compartments to survive a head-on collision, but not the sideswipe that happened when the helmsman tried to swerve.

It wasn't the fault of the nearby ship that failed to respond, or the Titanic radioman who ignored an iceberg warning early in the evening, or the one who later sent a wrong SOS position.

It was all those people's fault.

But it was *even more* the fault of something less tangible, and not a person at all: the overall *company culture* of the White Star Line that owned the Titanic. The beautiful, glorious Titanic sank on her maiden voyage because the White Star Line, *as a company,* was too highly focused on luxury and speed, at the expense of safety.

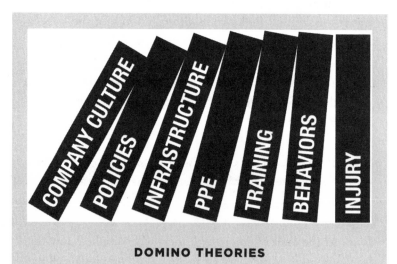

DOMINO THEORIES

What common chain of events leads to an accident? Back in 1931, safety researcher Herbert Heinrich proposed a famous domino theory of accident creation.[65] His first domino was "social environment and ancestry" followed by "fault of the person" and then "mechanical or physical hazard." That never worked for me. Above you can see a revised domino theory, in which the overall company culture is the first domino to fall, the piece that takes down all the rest.

HOW DO YOU TURN THE TITANIC?

In the introduction, I talked about good companies, bad companies, and companies trying to improve. If you are trying to turn your own Titanic, how do you proceed? How can someone at the top of an organizational chart—or halfway down—turn a great big heavy organization with hundreds, or thousands, or even tens of thousands of employees?

In 2004, David White became the global VP of the supply chain at Campbell's Soup Company. When he walked in the door, the company had a lost-time injury rate of 1.24.[66] That meant that of the 24,000 people working at Campbell's on any given day, an average of one person a day would be seriously injured or hurt, somewhere around the world. By the time White left ten years later, lost-time injuries had been reduced by 90 percent—with an average of two per month, down from the staggering thirty per month when he arrived.[67]

How did he do it? He changed the company culture.

Within days of starting his job, White sent a personal letter to every Campbell's plant and warehouse manager worldwide. In that letter he declared that: 1) he intended to cut lost-time injuries by 50 percent within three years; and 2) anytime a manager had a lost-time injury, they had to send him an email within twenty-four hours explaining what happened, how the person was doing, and what could be learned from the incident.

With these letters, and with his relentless follow-up, White declared that he was *turning the ship*. He made it clear that he cared *personally and deeply* about safety. That safety was his top priority. He did experience some pushback from managers who thought that such a dramatic reduction was impossible—and he spent a lot of time on the phone getting them onboard. Indeed, at one point the phone company revoked his phone card because it became suspicious of so many calls placed to Indonesia, Australia, and Mexico within one twenty-four-hour period.

Little by little, however, the entire company came around. Little by little, a new culture of safety took hold—and the results spoke for themselves. Protocols were changed. Infrastructure was adjusted. On-the-floor behaviors were modified. It all mattered.

If a lookout needed binoculars, damn it, binoculars were found.

White didn't just use sticks, he used carrots. He celebrated every reduction in lost-work injury rates, invited newspaper reports, put up festive safety flags, and added safety to the company's success scorecards. Recently, when asked what drove his efforts, White said, "In the end, if you reduce injury, your worker's compensation costs come down. But that's not what's driving you. What is? Your love for people, your caring about the organization, your caring about individuals. It's a big thing. People feeling like their company cares about their safety."[68]

NOT A PRIORITY...A PRECONDITION

Here's another discussion about company culture from retired Alcoa CEO Paul O'Neill, who I cannot help but quote at length:[69]

"For me, it's an element of a broader [philosophy] about human beings. In an organization that has the potential for greatness, [it should be] possible every day for every human being in that enterprise to say yes to three questions, without reservations. The first question, 'Are you treated with dignity and respect every day by everyone you encounter?' Question number two is, 'Are you given the things you need—tools, equipment, training, encouragement—so that you can make a contribution?' And three, 'Do you get the recognition you want for what you do?' Our human beings are our most important asset, but in most places, there's no proof it's really true. It's just something that is said.

"Safety should never be a priority. It should be a precondition, like before you can get up and walk around, you have to breathe. Safety should be like breathing. It's a precondition for organizational behavior. It's important that every person is valued and every injury is the responsibility of the whole organization and every manager."

When he left Alcoa, O'Neill was asked, "Were you a success?" Certainly, he was a resounding success in every area: in financial growth, stockholder value, and safety. But his answer concerned long-term company culture: "If the lost-work data and total recordable rate continue to fall long after I'm gone, I will have been a success."

WHAT IS A "SAFETY CULTURE"?

Before you try to turn the Titanic, you need to know where you want to head. You also need to know where you are.

How can you define the safety culture of a company? We'll talk about systems of hazard assessment, characteristics of attitude, internal social forces, commitment, and much more. At the end of the chapter, I'll even draw a pretty graphic. Ultimately, however, your safety culture boils down to this:

What is considered normal at this company?

If it's considered normal for people to suffer hand cuts on a near-daily basis, that attitude will be reflected in a thousand small decisions on policies, training, PPE, costs, infrastructure, and the hiring of work team supervisors. If it's normal to have a low rate of injury, with each event a significant occurrence, that too will be reflected in a thousand, day-to-day choices by management and workers alike.

How do the workers interact with each other when it comes to safety? Do they have each other's backs, reminding their coworkers to put on their gloves if they see someone not wearing theirs? And how does that coworker respond? With a rolling of the eyes or with a grateful nod? Once again, it all depends on what's considered normal.

Here's a similar definition I like:

A safety culture is how an organization behaves when no one is watching.

Either way, the meaning of "safety culture" goes way, way

beyond anything defined by government regulations. Both David White and Paul O'Neill *redefined normal* at their companies. If you are a CEO, or if you are a safety manager, or if you wield any influence at all, *that is your job too.*

Embrace it.

SEEING THE REALITY GAP

Understanding where your Titanic sits on the ocean partly means seeing the "reality gap" between official policy and the actual, on the ground actions of management and workers. Nothing is more important than the reality gap, particularly at a large company with lots of official policy. Are written policies *actually* enforced? Is the listed safety equipment *actually* available? Are the mandatory training sessions *actually* attended? Are checkoff lists reflecting *actual* inspections?

Once again: How do people behave when no one is watching?

Upper management often has a hard time seeing the reality gap in their own companies. If decisions are being made in a remote head office, it's easy to assume those decisions are actually being implemented on the ground. It's often hard to see how official policies, or the records kept during official inspections, deviate from what is actually normal on the ground.

If you are a CEO, or if you are a safety manager, or if you wield any influence at all, *clearly seeing the reality gap is another part of your job.*

DUPONT TURNED THEIR SHIP

The history of DuPont offers the perfect case study of a company that went from a poor safety culture to one of the most admired safety cultures in the world. Back in the early 1800s, when the DuPont family began making things like gunpowder, the workers developed a common expression, "That guy went across the creek."[70] This meant that the plant had blown up—again—and some poor worker had literally been blasted across the Brandywine River in Delaware where they were located. So common were these explosions that DuPont made the wall closest to the river out of wood instead of stone, so that wall would blow out, the building wouldn't collapse...and yes, people would "go across the river" where they had at least some chance of survival. In the DuPont Museum, you can see the blow-out wall preserved.

In 1817, seventy-seven-year-old Pierre Samuel DuPont died fighting a fire in the plant. In 1818, forty workers were killed, along with children in a school built on the grounds. By 1912, DuPont started collecting safety statistics, and by the 1990s they had set a goal of *zero* injuries.[71]

To achieve its present-day safety record, DuPont developed an almost unbelievably strict set of safety controls for chemical manufacture, with ironclad policies for every task performed by workers. As a result, not only are they famous for nearly eliminating the "reality gap" between policy and real action, but they now consult on safety to other companies. One of my colleagues who worked at DuPont (now merged with Dow Chemical), called the culture "weirdly, but wonderfully obsessed with protocol."

"In DuPont," wrote Winston P. Ledet, a former operations manager at the company, "we recognized that safety was the responsibility of each individual and required the participation of everyone." Thus the unique DuPont slogan: "Safety, I have to do it myself, but I can't do it alone."[72] It's a weird, but wonderful statement on how to do safety right.

It took multiple generations, but DuPont changed the definition of "normal" in their entire industry.

CAN YOU DO IT WITHOUT UPPER MANAGEMENT?

David White and Paul O'Neill were company officers with tremendous power to create change. So was the DuPont family. Can change be created without upper management? Could the Titanic have been turned by some responsible junior officer? Can hand safety become a company-wide priority through the efforts of a low-level manager?

The short answer is no.

I wish I could tell you otherwise, but study after study has shown that safety initiatives driven by any layer below top management generally fail to produce substantial and lasting results.[73] You can make limited progress on limited initiatives, but usually not the culture change that's really needed. People say, "Okay, this is going to last so long, then the safety manager will get canned or the budget's gonna get cut. I don't need to pay attention."

Indeed, changes in the overall safety culture of a company seem to require *a personal* belief and commitment on the part of top brass. Not just a logical decision. That personal commitment may *begin* with a logical decision based on worker's comp costs, lost-time analyses, lawsuits, or government regulation. But at some point, it has to reach the gut. The company officers have to *care* at an emotional level.

Otherwise, the entire company senses the lack of commitment, and a true safety culture never develops.

The Challenges to Caring

There are two significant challenges anyone faces when trying to engage upper management personally in this issue.

The first is the psychological gulf between upper management and workers, in that upper managers usually are not physically at risk in the workplace. Yes, it's that simple. Often managers have never actually quite "been there" and felt the risks, while workers feel personally vulnerable every single day. Subconsciously, the brain may say, "If it could happen to me, I care; but if I am personally safe, I am allowed to care a little less." No one may say such an awful thing aloud, but the feeling may be there.

This gulf also leads to a kind of organizational blindness. Indeed, a 2015 study of management vs. worker perceptions of company culture showed that again and again, managers viewed their safety culture as much more sound than their workers.[74]

Secondly, whenever management looks at the issue, it will always see a perceived trade-off between productivity and safety—whether that trade-off is real or not. Management at all levels has a tremendous incentive to increase productivity, and only a personal commitment to safety has any chance of overcoming that bias.

Here's the truth: shortcuts *can* lead to speed, but the truth is, people in safe organizations are overwhelmingly more productive on a long-term basis. This has been proven time and time again. For example, Steve Ludwig, currently the safety manager at Rockwell Automation, found that Best in Class companies—those that score in the top 20 percent of aggregate performance scores—were also the companies exhibiting the lowest injury frequency rate. In fact, their injury frequency of 0.05 percent was eighteen times better than average and sixty times better than the worst performers.[75]

WHAT DRIVES A PERSONAL COMMITMENT FROM UPPER MANAGEMENT?

Ledcor is a major Canadian construction company which has won many awards for safety. What created this commitment? A personal tragedy. Founder William Lede died in 1980 when a gravel pile collapsed on him at a jobsite. When his sons Dave and Herb took over, the memory of that day created a personal passion for job safety.[76] It's worth reading Ledcor's impressive safety poster:

LEDCOR SAFETY COMMITMENTS
THINK SAFETY WORK SAFELY
We think safety and work safely by caring for each other.

I DO MY JOB SAFELY.
No job is so urgent or important that it cannot be done safely.

WE WORK TOGETHER TO IMPROVE SAFETY.
We work with our fellow employees, our contractors, and partners to share ideas and develop "next" practices—always going forward together.

WE TAKE CARE OF EACH OTHER.
If I take care of myself and others, business will take care of itself.

WE FOCUS ON PREVENTION.
Through the implementation of our health and safety program, we can prevent incidents and stop people from getting hurt.

I PLAN MY WORK FOR SAFE PRODUCTION.
I use HS&E tools and training to plan my work safely.

I ACT WHEN THERE'S SOMETHING UNSAFE.
I intervene, correct, or speak up about any health and safety issue.

I BELIEVE IN SAFETY, ALL THE TIME.
Safety is on-the-job, off-the-job, and everywhere in between.

As a worker, contractor, manager, or visitor, you are demonstrating your personal commitment to Ledcor's Health, Safety & Environmental Protection Policy and Program. Thank you for your support and belief that zero incidents through best practices is possible.

HOW TO GET A CEO TO CARE

It's an urban myth that "no one changes until they hit rock bottom." A CEO does not have to see a tragic industrial accident in their family or be standing at a jobsite when a worker loses a hand to find a personal commitment to safety. If you are a CEO reading this book, I certainly hope nothing like that happens to you.

Still, a change of heart does seem to require a *moment of realization*, when a person says, "Okay, I am going to change. I am going to make this my priority."

Contrary to popular belief, that moment does not generally come from looking at a bunch of ROI graphs comparing the costs of safety versus a reduction in worker's compensation costs—though such graphs certainly count. CEOs are not robots, they're human beings. Dollars and cents are motivators, but not really the top motivators of their behavior. Indeed, plenty of studies have shown that *all* major human decisions are more emotional than logical. The emotion comes first; the logic just backs it up.[77]

What follows are some concrete steps a safety manager can take to get upper management to take safety to heart.

MAKE STATS PERSONAL

Start making hand safety a personal issue for upper management by including the real life stories of injured workers in reports.

Don't just report: "We had five hand injuries last month, with one significant lost-time injury."

Instead, spell it out personally. "We had five injuries last month, including Bill Thompson, whose hand was crushed in a conveyor belt in the Arcadia plant. Bill has been out for two weeks, and has already had two surgeries. It's uncertain when and if he can return to work. Bill is thirty-two, and he has a wife and two kids under age five. We are investigating, but it's clear that someone disabled the proximity alert on the belt because it kept going off with false alarms. Bill's wife is June, and her phone number is XXX-XXX-XXXX. The supervisor of that unit is Gabe Turner."

Even better would be to get the CEO to personally deliver the safety report as part of upper management meetings.

If the CEO tells the story of Bill Thompson, it will matter a great deal more to both the CEO and to his managers.

DRIVE THE UNDERSTANDING THAT ONLY MANAGEMENT CAN CREATE SAFETY

Often you will find a mistaken impression among managers that only workers can watch out for their own safety. This is patently untrue, of course, but the following story may help illustrate the issue.

I often think about the story of a worker who had long-term nerve damage from HAVS, hand-arm vibration syndrome, from working with pneumatic drills. He'd drive home with numb hands, but not even think about it, and he'd worry about picking things up safely at home. When the company finally gave him the right kind of gloves to protect against the vibration of tools, *at the age when he had already become a grandfather,* he did slowly improve and he wept when he was finally able to safely hold his grandchild.[78]

Here's what I think when I remember that story: *This worker never would have figured out HAVS or found the right anti-vibration gloves on his own.* You have to know there is such a thing as HAVS. You have to know about the special gloves, and you have to have them provided long term and kept in good condition. Only management can ensure that all their workers have this knowledge and wear these gloves when using pneumatic tools.

Only management has the big view, so only management can mitigate certain risks. How can you get upper management to realize this at your company? And then see the results?

FRAME SAFETY AS RELATIONSHIP BUILDING

Paul O'Neill realized early on in his tenure at Alcoa that a focus on safety was a sure way to build a strong relationship between management and workers. *Nothing better showed workers that management cared.* Nothing better contributed to morale. With good morale comes productivity, creativity, and a willingness to pitch in when needed.

A discussion about safety forms an immediate emotional bond with anyone. You can throw a hundred company picnics. You can give out a thousand "best employee" awards. You can give Christmas turkeys and annual bonuses. But nothing says you care like walking the line and talking to the workers about their *safety*—then doing something about it.

In short, management must learn that safety is a key ingredient in long-term success.

Could you get the CEO to see hand safety as a way to connect to workers?

START SMALL

Don't launch your effort to win over management with a huge, fully thought-out safety initiative that includes comprehensive hazard assessments, new gloves, signs, training programs, and all the other good stuff we advocate in this book.

Get your foot in the door with something small, something that sets the pattern, shows immediate feel-good results, and starts to change upper management culture.

Something like: "I'd like to try upgrading the signage on the main floor to show the safe way to do things and not just give a bunch of vague warnings (see chapter five on doing this right). I'd like to see if that reduces hand injuries. The cost will be minimal." Then, a couple months later: "The rate of injuries we get in the cutting room is pretty high. I'd like to try out these new cut-resistant Kevlar models, at least on a pilot basis."

You will be setting a pattern, and upper management will start seeing itself as a positive actor in changing the safety culture at your company. The COO and CEO will start seeing themselves as *the kind of person who does these kinds of things* for their workers. It will become part of their identity. Eventually, you can spring your complete plan on them.

What small step could you propose which would be immediately acceptable to upper management?

THE POWER OF PUBLIC COMMITMENT

If you can get your upper managers to speak publicly about safety, in speeches to workers, in a published op-ed, or at an industry conference, it can go a long way to creating personal commitment. People do feel accountable for their own words to others, spoken in public. They begin to internalize the ideas they have expressed, and they want to live up to their public statements.

Suppose you help draft a speech for your CEO to give at a company meeting or a conference?

The same is true at the worker level, by the way. If you can get workers to speak publicly, in a group meeting, about how to be safe, it's much more likely they will follow through when the situation arises.

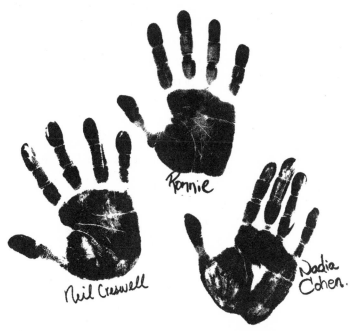

At the Rio Tinto mine in Northern Quebec, both managers and workers were asked to put their handprints on a board outside the mine and sign their names next to their prints. The board read "I'm Committed to Hand Safety."

Bottom line? This public commitment helped drive down injury rates.

THE POWER OF WRITING THINGS DOWN

Door-to-door salespeople selling things like encyclopedias,

vacuum cleaners, and insurance know a simple trick to lower the rates of contract cancellations after the customer has had a chance to cool off. The salesperson asks the customer to fill out the contract themselves, instead of the salesperson filling in the blanks.

There's something extremely powerful in the act of writing something down. It creates a whole different level of emotional obligation. If you can get your CEO and other managers to physically write down their goals for safety, say reducing lost-time hand injuries below 1 percent, it can go a long way to keeping up their commitment over time.

Could you propose language for the CEO to write into a communication sent from their personal email?

SELF-ASSEMBLY BUILDS ENGAGEMENT

People place far more value on things they have helped construct. If you go to upper management with a fully conceived hand-safety plan, it is much less likely they will feel personally committed to that plan than if you work with them, over time, to create it.

Psychologists sometimes call this the "Ikea effect," after the furniture retailer that demands lots of self-assembly by its customers.[79] No middle manager should ever forget the Ikea effect.

A great way of engaging upper management is simply to ask for their advice. For example, ask the CEO for his or her input on safety training, or ask them to help customize the program by deciding which modules should be included.

How could you include upper managers in creating plans, even in a minor way?

SOCIAL PROOF CAUSES ACTION

Bartenders salt their tip jars with a few dollars to simulate tips left by prior customers, thus establishing social proof that tipping is normal. Workers will put on gloves if the workers around them put on gloves. CEOs will sponsor safety programs if they see other CEOs sponsoring safety programs.

Get the idea?

If you say, "I was talking to John Smith at Respected Competitor Inc., and he mentioned their injury rates are way down because of their new safety training program," it can go a long way to getting a training program going at your company, too.

Never say, "Some great new gloves have appeared on the market, let's try them out." Instead, say, "Most of the industry has moved on from leather gloves, including Respected Competitor Inc. We really should run a pilot with Kevlar."

Don't say, "I want to look into getting better safety guards for that equipment." Instead say, "It's become standard practice to refit this kind of equipment with better, after-market guards. I think we need to get up to speed on that."

What research can you do on practices in your industry and at your competitors, so you are prepared to reframe the conversation with upper management?

SHOW THAT *YOU* CARE ABOUT OTHER ISSUES THAN SAFETY

Too often I've seen health and safety experts who put on blinders and refuse to acknowledge the goals and priorities of other departments. If you want the attention of managers at any level you have to acknowledge their focus on productivity and controlling costs. Yes, health and safety should be a precondition for work, but it's hardly the only issue facing management.

Whenever you discuss safety, you need to show that you are on the team. You need to listen to all the problems facing managers and you need to make sure you don't isolate yourself from these problems.

As an HSE, you need to build the same kind of personal relationships as everyone else in the company. That may include especially purchasing managers. Do someone a favor and they will do you a favor. Ask them for a favor (see the sidebar on the Franklin Effect), and that will help, too. Find a common bond and that bond may prove critical to the health and well-being of everyone. That's how humans have always operated, and how they always will. You can't stand outside the company conversation, yelling about safety.

Ask a purchasing manager to take some different gloves home and try them out. Get their advice. If you can get a lower price on some equipment, save your moment. Go to the PM and say, "Hey, we're buying these safety vests, but I found this lower price. What do you think?"

You will have just made a new friend.

USE THE BEN FRANKLIN EFFECT

Maybe you've heard of a psychological phenomenon called the "Ben Franklin Effect." It's counterintuitive, but true—and a great tool for any safety manager to win people over. A fellow legislator in Pennsylvania hated old Ben. In order to bring this rival around, Franklin asked if he could borrow a rare and valuable book from his rival's library. The gentleman found this flattering and lent the book willingly. Franklin dutifully returned the book just a week later with a nice thank-you note. He never even read it.

Result? The gentleman didn't hate Franklin anymore, and began to cooperate on new legislation.

A psychological study in 1969[80] proved the Franklin Effect true by finding that in general, we like people better who have asked us for favors. Why? According to researchers, that's because we subconsciously can't reconcile hating someone with the fact that we did them a favor. Also, we assume that someone who asks for a favor likes us, and subconsciously, we want to reciprocate.[81] Asking for a favor also simply reduces the personal distance between people. This makes it imperative not to use an intermediary, and to always make the request in person.

Can you use the Ben Franklin Effect to overcome barriers between yourself and a manager, or yourself and workers? Try it. Ask for a favor and see what happens.

FINALLY, YES, ROI COUNTS

In this section we've talked about getting a personal commitment from CEOs and other upper management. But yes, of course, ROI demonstrations matter, too.

There are plenty of case studies on the way safety initiatives substantially cut costs in worker's compensation, lost time, and turnover—and typically, each dollar invested in injury prevention returns between two dollars and six dollars[82]—but those case studies are really only relevant within your particular industry.

For example, we had a large automobile tire retailer who was spending fifty cents a pair on gloves and we worked with them to design a much better glove that cost them fourteen dollars a pair. Their annual glove costs shot up by $200,000, but at the end of the year, their own cost analysis said they had saved over $1 million overall. How? Their worker's comp costs dropped. Their lost-time costs dropped. Most importantly, their turnover rate dropped by 10 percent, and that alone saved them a fortune on recruiting, training, and lost-time costs. Indeed, the improved gloves increased dexterity to the point that they actually sped up production.

Not to mention, of course, that workers experienced far fewer injuries.

What specific case studies can you find for your particular industry, to bolster your safety arguments to management? What case studies within your own company?

INJURIES COST EVERYONE, BIG TIME

Sam Cunard is a veteran safety manager. He tells a lot of stories about the meaning of "ROI" in different places he has worked. "Cuts and bruises and abrasions and blisters and punctures and wounds to the hands. They happen. You go to a manager and you say, 'Listen, let's start giving these people gloves.' The manager replies, "Do you know what gloves cost?' I reply, 'Do you know what three stitches cost? More than three stitches, that's what. People go on antibiotics, the antibiotics don't work, they get infected, then they're in pain so they go on oxycontin—it goes on and on. I just documented a case where a guy cut his hand in California, and didn't report it. He got a splinter in his hand that never healed, and the wound eventually ended up getting MRSA and his hand had to be amputated. To make matters worse, because he didn't report it, he couldn't prove that the accident happened at work, so he couldn't get worker's comp to pay for it. All because he had no gloves."

This was a disaster for the worker, but also for his work team, for the morale of the company.

How do you convey that kind of ROI analysis to management?

HOW TO REACH WORKERS

So far we've talked about managing up. Now, what about managing down?

It's surprisingly difficult to get workers involved in safety initiatives. It's even harder to shift worker cultures. As we have learned, humans feel most comfortable doing things the way they have always been done, even if that way is dangerous.

If you are a safety manager, however, it's your job to get workers *deeply* involved and to *substantially* shift their attitudes about safety. It's just not enough to do "what's possible in this environment and with workers who think this way."

What if that lookout on the Titanic had refused to go on duty until somebody broke open the locker containing the binoculars?

What if one worker at your company said to another, "Hey, I'm not going into that pit with you unless you put on your gloves."

Farfetched? I'm hoping not.

FIGHTING TRIBALISM

As in all areas of life, birds of a feather flock together in the workplace. Too often, people only really interact with others who are in their department, workgroup, or organization level. Managers consult with managers. Workers talk amongst themselves. Tribalism runs rampant at all levels.

But safety, more than any other workplace issue, requires extensive cooperation between all the cultures and subcultures in a company. There's just no other way to make safety happen. Changing worker attitudes requires changing management attitudes first, then overcoming tribalism as managers work to make improvements. That means opening up the conversation.

Before you decide what's hand-safe for workers, it's plain common sense to ask the workers what they think. What's the best PPE? The most comfortable gloves? The right protocol? They're the experts, right? They're the ones who are going to have to wear those gloves, no?

Far too often, however, such decisions are made at the management or purchasing level without consulting workers at all. In my business, I see that mistake made every single day. *When workers are not involved, not only do wrongheaded decisions get made, but it becomes extremely difficult to get worker buy-in, even if you have chosen the right course.*

To engage workers, you have to move from sermons to discussions, from PowerPoint shows to structured conversations. As we will see in chapter eight, all training must also include these discussions and enable easy feedback. Or it just won't work.

IF YOU DON'T HELP FORMULATE A RULE, YOU FOLLOW IT ONLY WHEN THE RULEMAKER IS WATCHING

When we asked safety expert, Timothy Ludwig, about involving people at the worksite in hand-safety decisions, he got a bit worked up on the issue: "You ask questions! You ask them! If you tell employees to do stuff, they'll do it when you're around. If you ask them and the decision is made or the policies or whatever are based on their decisions, they're more likely to do it. It's quite a simple principle. You come up with it yourself, you've got to follow your own rules, right?...My definition [of a good safety culture] is people talking to each other. If PPE is just, 'Here, you must wear these. It's the rule. If you get caught without wearing them, you're in trouble,' you're going through the dysfunctional practices that will only get you a *little bit* of compliance."

A little bit of compliance is not enough.

LEARNING THE HACKS

If you involve workers by asking them questions and allowing them to test out new safety products before they're forced to use them, you will not only get their buy-in, you will learn their personal "safety hacks." Don't undervalue these personal hacks: maybe everyone could learn something from them.

Safety expert, Timothy Ludwig, notes a worker who always put his gloves on top of his safety boots in his locker at the end of the day, so he would put them on as a matter of course after he tied his boots.[83] Simple, but effective—and why not suggest that to others?

Another hack was to always have several extra pairs of gloves at a worksite, since gloves are so often lost or damaged. Obvious and simple, right? But that's exactly the kind of crucial, unofficial hack that makes all the difference.

A third, great hack involved the grip on gloves. At a helicopter manufacturer, they were using cut-resistant gloves with a lot of grip, but for a certain part of the job they wanted no grip—they needed to run their hands across the blade to ensure it was finished properly. The solution? Turn the glove inside out. Now it had the same cut protection, but no grip.

Ludwig calls these "b-hacks," for behavior-based safety hacks.

It's hard to learn b-hacks from people unless you engage them regularly, make them believe you prioritize safety, and show that you actually care to learn from them.

It has to be an ongoing dialog, however. Not a once a year event.

That makes it doubly the responsibility of the safety manager to keep the conversation afloat.

HOW DO YOU MAKE IT ABOUT THE TEAM?

Everybody knows that team spirit is vital to safety. People have to watch each other's backs. People have to remind each other to do things safely. People have to feel comfortable pointing out issues.

That means that workers have to feel that they and their bosses are all in it together. This is a huge challenge.

Team spirit doesn't just happen, you have to make it happen, especially given the huge diversity of workforces, and the natural barriers between management and labor. Supervisors have to specifically say, out loud, like an athletic coach, "We all have to care that everybody's okay at the end of the day. I care, and I need all of you to care about each other. See something, say something, save someone. We are all in this together."

They have to mean it. And then they have to put on their gloves, too.

I'm not going to go into specific team-building exercises—you'll find plenty of books with great ideas for team building. I'll just say that such exercises are not stupid or unnecessary. No matter how artificial they may seem at first, they work, partly because they just get people to talk to each other in a more open way.

The safety manager can be key to team building—again, partly because nothing creates more of a personal connection than talking about safety. I have watched many safety managers at work, both in person and in training videos, and the best share this trait: *They are firm, but friendly.* They joke around, they show genuine concern, but they never bend on the rules. And they are never afraid to point out issues, to anyone, at any time. *That sets the model for everyone to follow, top to bottom.*

TOM VS. DARRYL

I often think about the words of safety expert Timothy Ludwig, when he discusses meeting two different styles of safety manager, who he names Tom and Darryl:[84]

> ...I was walking around with Tom at a steel smelting plant taking a tour of the fiery cauldron of hell that produces the lava flows that end up as posts for our road signs. I spent the day with an employee team charged with rolling out and managing their behavioral safety program. Tom was their safety manager and champion...On the tour Tom was pointing out hazards he wanted to fix and impartially talking about the most prominent risks at the plant. But what caught my attention was how the folks in different parts of the plant lit up when he walked in with me. Tom had intentionally associated his presence with a pleasant experience every time he interacted with his workers. He smiled, called them by name, asked about their kids or motorcycle, and always praised them for something they were doing to make the plant safer. And for that, when he asked for suggestions or had to discuss some at-risk behaviors, he generally got a lot of interaction, even if it was a hard topic to discuss. He always left with a smile, a thumbs-up, and "thanks." As we walked toward his workers they would smile and relax, even when talking about hazards or inspection results.

> ...Darryl (the name has been changed) took me around his elec-

tronic parts plant in Arizona. Darryl had a cramped little office full of safety reward swag and looked overwhelmed with all the work he had to do...I was struck by how workers reacted when he entered their space. I could see heads turning to see who was coming and then quickly turning back to their work. Some supervisors hurriedly stashed paperwork and others who were taking a break quickly returned to their task. When Darryl and I walked up to workers I saw their shoulders arch up to their ears as their bodies tightened. Others grimaced as if a sour stomach cramped up...No one wanted to start a conversation.

"How did Tom and Darryl elicit these different responses from workers? Over time their behavior while interacting with their workers shaped an automatic response.

I ask you, who do you think got more done, hand-safety-wise?

OVERCOMING THE GAPS THAT DESTROY TEAM SPIRIT

I've said that safety requires all the levels of a company working closely together—more than in any other issue a company faces. We've already discussed some of the gaps that make it so hard to get management and workers on the same team. What can be done about these gaps in your company? Let's list them.

Experience Gap: Managers often have no hands-on experience doing the work. Workers know that, so they don't listen to management safety advice or policies. *Great managers, and even CEOs, must get out on the line and actually do the work at least once, to understand it and develop credibility.* Not to mention empathy. As a manager myself, I try never to forget this great truth. Indeed, my father drilled it into me. When I was a teenager starting out in the family glove business, he told me I had to start at the bottom—and on one of my first days, I was sent down into the leather sludge pit, where all the waste went down. I'd be down there shoveling sludge for hours, where the smell was overpowering. Trust me, I never forgot that *someone had to do that job. It was tough. And it was dangerous.*

Risk Gap: Managers do not face the same risks as workers. *Along with experiencing the work at least once, specific personal empathy for injuries must be shown by management. Make that phone call after an injury!*

Budget Silos: Purchasing tries to save money on gloves and other PPE in a materials budget. Managers try to reduce costs and increase output under a production budget. Fines and worker's comp claims may not directly impact either of these budgets, leading to false economies at the expense of worker safety. PMs and managers get their bonuses even though injuries are bleeding both workers and ledgers. *Great COOs and CEOs make sure that intelligent accounting make for true ROI across budget silos.*

Reality Gap: Policies are announced but not enforced. Statistics don't reflect reality. Promised changes and equipment never materialize. Managers typically think the work is being performed far more safely than it really is—and workers always know the difference. *Great managers completely eliminate reality gaps.*

When these reality gaps become too glaring, trust disappears—and teams are all about trust. No trust, no team.

How do you know you have a genuine team spirit happening? When anyone on the team feels comfortable sharing anything with anyone else on the team, including team leaders.

Creating that comfort can be extremely challenging—I won't sugarcoat it. National culture may stand against it. The management/worker gaps in the sidebar may stand against it. Generation gaps may stand against it—lately, for example, baby boomers and millennials may not respect each other as they should. The particular people and their histories may stand against it.

But let me repeat: nothing can cut through barriers better than a mutual concern for safety, stated clearly, with discussion and feedback, every single day.

Along the way, every discussion has to be framed as "It's all our job to protect each other," never "This is just the rule, so follow it." Frame the discussion poorly, and when you punish someone for not following protocol, you will unintentionally communicate not safety concerns, but fear: "Don't report things or your buddies will get punished."

HOW CAN YOU CHANGE NORMS AT THE WORKER LEVEL?

If everyone around you is wearing gloves and acting safely, odds are you will too, just because it seems like the normal thing to do. Newcomers are influenced by the frequency, uniformity, and consistency of what they observe in their first few days—and then the pattern is set, for better or for worse.[85]

How do you change long-established, but dangerous norms? Here are some proven approaches.

Create a Larger Frame of Reference

If you go to a shop floor where no one has ever worn gloves to do their work, and you say, "We just bought all these beautiful, cut-resistant gloves. You need to start wearing them to improve safety around here," you will probably be met with shrugs. A week later, the gloves will be forgotten.

It's much better to say, "We have a lot of hand injuries, but our competitors, including Acme Metal Fabricators down the street, are wearing these gloves and they have way fewer injuries. We're not up to the norm for our industry. We're not doing what everyone else does out there."

Not, "we have to act differently," but "we have to act normally." Basic human psychology.

Introduce New Policies with Clear Reasons and Demonstrations

Workers are adults. Like you, they don't take to rules that don't make sense to them. In fact, let me say something you may find irritating: *If people don't follow rules, it's your fault as management, not their fault as workers. You didn't explain it right. You didn't enforce it right. You didn't get them on board.*

We already talked about the importance of involving workers in safety decisions, but at some point, a new policy has to be locked down and enforced. When that happens, it's your job to get people on board as adults.

Don't say, "Here's the new lockout/tagout policy for the electrical equipment. Thanks to everyone who came to the meetings and contributed to figuring this out."

Instead say, "As you know, we've had some injuries from people handling equipment when they didn't know it was left on by the last guy. It's not an easy problem to solve, but thanks to everyone who came to the meetings, we went through a lot of different options. Today we are officially starting the new lockout/tagout policy on equipment. Yes, it's something of a hassle, but I'm confident, and everyone who contributed ideas is confident, that it's the best option for ensuring the safety of the hands and fingers of everyone you work with. If everyone follows this protocol, we're going to have a lot fewer injuries, so we're going to be tough in enforcing it. But we need your support and cooperation to do it right."

Then demonstrate the new policies, hands-on—no matter how simple and obvious they may seem. Walk to the machine, and tag it out. Better yet, have a worker demo the action.

Establish Clear Safety Roles within Teams

There's a famous saying: "If everyone is responsible then no one is responsible." This saying's just not true when it comes to safety, because *everyone* is responsible for safety—but it does make for good organizational thinking.

If you introduce a new policy like the lockout/tagout policy above, it's much better if you also say, "Tom here has volunteered to be the lockout/tagout monitor. He's going to keep his eye out, and if anyone's doing this wrong or forgetting to do it at all, he's going to come up and remind you."

Another worker could be the glove monitor—making sure everyone has and wears the right gloves.

Now, certainly the team lead or supervisor needs to have the ultimate responsibility for policy enforcement. Tom is not going to be at fault if the policy isn't followed. But involving workers in this way can go a long way toward breaking down barriers and establishing new team norms.

SAFETY CHAMPIONS AND WORKER-LEVEL TASK FORCES

You can go beyond ad hoc safety roles within a single work team by establishing a volunteer "safety champion." This person maintains safety checklists, identifies issues, and takes on a formal advisory role on behalf of the team to management or a company-wide safety committee.

The safety champion can receive additional training and be responsible for training new team members, but it's important that this person does not become "management," is not evaluated on the basis of their safety work, and does not bear responsibility for results. They have to remain workers who merely advocate for safety and encourage safety within the team, otherwise their credibility will be questioned.

If you find a volunteer to be safety champion, make sure it's someone with deep experience and respect within the team. Choosing a respected, highly skilled champion will in itself help create new norms within the group.

One company has reported success with "safety task forces" entirely drawn from workers. These task forces cut across work disciplines, meet every other week, do hazard assessments, and come up with specific safety initiatives in cooperation with management.

Worker-led efforts, encouraged by management, go a long way toward building trust and establishing new team norms. These efforts can be led by a safety champion.

WRONG WAYS AND RIGHT WAYS TO CREATE POLICY

Hand safety requires hand-safety policies. But as we saw with the "reality gap," arbitrary or unenforced policies are not only meaningless, they give a false impression of safety to upper management, and create scorn and distrust among workers.

Far too often, policies are developed by managers working in a vacuum—or rather, in a remote highrise—using cut-and-paste industry policies or expensive consultants who have never spoken to the workers on the ground. Far too often, there's no follow-up to see if specific policies are actually reducing injuries.

Go back and read that sidebar on the gaps between management and workers to see how destructive such an approach can be to overall trust and the safety culture of a company.

Importantly, policies have to apply to management as well as to workers, and must clearly put responsibilities on both. Here are the unavoidable steps. Don't be tempted to skip any of them.

1. Research the baseline safety standards and hazard issues for your specific industry. Know what others are doing and

how it is working for them. There's no excuse for not doing this homework, but it is often neglected.

2. Understand the psychology of safety we discussed in chapter three.

3. Identify specific hazards. Set up a process for ongoing identification of hazards—it's not a one-time thing. Involve workers and use chapter seven of this book to guide you.

4. Develop written policies, programs, and processes in cooperation with worker safety champions and safety committees. Policies must be written down in simple, clear language, available to anyone.

5. Do the infrastructure work described in chapter five. This includes signage, etc., right at the worksite. *Policy must not be used to cover up bad infrastructure.*

6. Educate, educate, educate. Managers and workers must be trained and retrained as policies are rolled out. See chapter eight for how to do training right.

7. Rigorously investigate and report all accidents and injuries, then follow up with policy, infrastructure, and training changes. Be totally open about these changes and why they occur. If there's no feedback loop between incidents and policies, the "reality gap" will continue to build, and trust will be lost.

8. Keep the right metrics and actually use those metrics in a feedback loop to adjust policies and improve safety. Do this on a regular schedule. Read chapter nine on the whole issue of good vs. worthless metrics.

Overall, remember this wonderful saying: *Policies are the management of uncertainty.* Policies are the way that groups of humans cope with the otherwise random forces of the universe. Everyone should see policies and protocols in that positive light: not bureaucracy, not CYA, but safety.

ENFORCEMENT

Policies without enforcement aren't policies, they're "guidelines." It's nice to be nice, but ultimately, safety must be nonnegotiable.

That means you have to use both carrots and sticks. Let's take a look at both.

Carrots

As we discussed under chapter two, mistake #3, it's easy to get safety incentives wrong. Carrots for correctly following policy cannot be "rewards for low rates of injuries," they have to be rewards for things like "taking safe actions" or "consistently wearing PPE." Indeed, it may be illegal to give rewards for low injury rates, because of the way you are incentivizing people not to report injuries.

Rewards can be divided into *financial rewards* and *social rewards*.

Financial Rewards

Financial rewards are the most obvious, and in some ways, the easiest to provide. But one problem with any kind of financial rewards is that they tend to produce only short-term results, while social rewards can create long-lasting change. In any case, financial rewards tend to be unpredictable, and studies are inconclusive.

For example, in one study, a group of smokers were told to try to quit cigarettes. All were given forty-five dollars a month to come in for each interview and blood draw, to see if they had really stopped. Incentive group members were additionally promised a $750 reward if they made it without smoking for six months. A tiny 9.4 percent of the incentive group made it six months, compared to just 3.6 percent of the control group. Fine. But another six months out, the results were reversed, and a significantly higher proportion of the incentive group had gone back to smoking.[86]

On the other hand, companies like Campbell Soup have reported good results from safety incentives which included monetary rewards.

Bottom line? Financial incentives for consistently safe *behaviors* (not statistics) can supplement an overall effort to change the safety culture in a company, but they cannot be the linchpin of those efforts.

Social Rewards

Social rewards in the form of praise and recognition for safe behaviors are, in general, far more effective than financial rewards. Indeed, social rewards are fundamental to any culture of safety. They create internal motivations, they build team spirit, and they show that management values workers more than it values money.

Social rewards can be as simple as a supervisor walking by and publicly praising someone for handling a machine properly, wearing their gloves consistently, or protecting a coworker. More formal recognition can come in weekly safety meetings or the like.

Either way, sooner is far better than later. Immediate positive feedback is much more meaningful to people than delayed feedback.

In a truly great safety culture, workers praise one another for safe behaviors. Everyone provides social rewards.

STICKS

Using sticks to enforce policy offers a tougher psychological problem. Here are some guidelines:

1. As discussed earlier, safety managers and inspectors must be firm but friendly. You must always convey the sense that all actions are taken to protect the team, and that everyone is in it together. Punishments should not be "management clamping down" but "the team looking out for its members." It's all in how you phrase it.

2. Inspections must not be predictable. Workers must always believe there's a chance of a manager appearing unexpectedly and observing a lack of safety. But as we discussed many times, the key to people acting safely even when no one is watching is to involve them in the process of developing the rules and keeping the rules relevant to the actual work.

3. Employees must have a clear understanding of penalties for failing to take precautions. No surprises. Surprises undermine trust.

4. Penalties must be given out consistently. Nothing makes a worker more angry than being punished for breaking a safety rule when another worker got off scot-free.

5. There cannot be any kind of punishment for a person who actually gets injured. This will lead to anger and to the covering up of incidents.

6. Consider all alternatives before applying discipline—positive reinforcement is always more effective than negative reinforcement.

7. Consequences have to be consistent and immediate. The

longer the time that passes, the less impact a consequence will have. If a supervisor chastises a worker a week after seeing an issue, he won't have nearly the impact of walking by and saying "Jack, you need to wear your gloves. Now."

THERE'S THE DOOR

When asked about enforcement, one safety manager told us this story:

"A supervisor called me and said, 'You have to come down to the floor. A worker is causing a storm yelling about being told to wear his gloves.' Sure enough, when I walk onto the floor, this guy is screaming because he's been written up twice in one night for not wearing his gloves. When I learned from the supervisor that the worker had been written up numerous times in the past for not wearing his gloves, I stood in front of everyone and said to the worker, very calmly, 'Hand me your keycard and head on out.'

"Word of this event spread quickly through the whole company. Everywhere I went, people would say, 'Is it true that this guy was let go for not wearing gloves?' I'd reply, calmly, 'Well, he's suspended pending termination, due to the number of write-ups he had about gloves.'

"As the night progressed, I began to see *everyone* wearing their gloves.

"I hate working that way. I'd rather say, 'Look, we want you to wear gloves so you don't get injured, not 'you don't wear

THE PROBLEM WITH PUBLIC SHAMING

Back in chapter two, mistake #4, we pointed out some of the problems with public shaming.

In the sidebar above, a worker is terminated publicly when he complains about wearing gloves. Notice, however, that the safety manager did not *shame* the worker. He did not say, "You're an idiot for not wearing gloves." He just calmly told the guy to turn in his keycard.

When giving penalties or corrections, you must always remember to focus on the act, not on the person.

You need to call out a person who is doing something unsafely or outside of policy, but it has to be in the context of protecting a valuable person and their valuable teammates. After being called out, a worker may feel guilty about breaking the rules and endangering others, but they should not feel *shame* or be called out for being a bad or inferior person. There's a huge difference.

When you *shame* a worker, you are inviting the resentment of all the workers. *You are separating yourself from the team.* Whatever the immediate impact of your harsh words, you are helping create a poor culture of safety overall.

CRYING "STOP WORK"

Are workers at your company empowered to call for work to stop if they see an unsafe condition? There may be no clearer measure of a mature safety culture than one where *anyone* feels comfortable exercising such a power. Is a safety shield broken? Were gloves not brought to the worksite? Is a machine suddenly displaying unsafe motions? Or is a worker simply unsure how to proceed safely, because inadequate instructions have been provided? If so, can he or she stand up and say, "I'm calling for a time-out until I understand how to proceed safely here."

The drilling crew at one major oil platform created a specific "Time Out for Safety" protocol, and made it clear that workers had an *obligation* to call a TOFS if an unsafe condition were observed or suspected.[87] At such a moment, of course, it's important that the task being performed be stopped safely— and a supervisor may decide it's safer to proceed than to stop at that point. But part of the deal is that the TOFS has to be acknowledged and received with a positive attitude.

No one can get angry at the worker calling the TOFS, even if it's called because the worker doesn't understand the plan, isn't clear what happens next, has a personal impairment, or sees that fewer people are involved in the task than originally scheduled.

Once a TOFS is called, everyone involved needs to agree on how to fix the problem and agree when it's fixed. When the ultimate work authority gives the all clear, that decision has to be documented.

A HAND SAFETY MATURITY MODEL

Many people have tried to define a "safety maturity model" for companies, but I have never seen one focused on hand safety. Let me offer my own, in the hope that it will help you see how far your company has come—and help you educate others. This one is slightly modified from the excellent maturity model created by the University of Queensland for the UK mining industry.[88]

I hope it brings this entire chapter into focus.

Importantly, the rungs on this ladder depend not on statistics, but on *attitude*. As we'll see in chapter nine, the right stats can be helpful, but they cannot show if you have created a true culture of safety. Why? Because a lack of injuries in the past is not necessarily indicative of a lack of injuries in the future. Remember again that BP's Deepwater Horizon had a near-perfect safety record before it blew up, killing eleven workers. The Titanic ran smoothly until it hit an iceberg.

Just as importantly, the model does not focus on compliance with safety regulations. In the US, for example, OSHA offers only vague direction on PPE for hands. Why? Because the dangerous tasks performed by workers with their hands are so incredibly varied, and change so often, and are so individual to particular companies, that it's impossible to create specific regulations.

SEEING WHAT'S NORMAL

As with all questions of culture, the model focuses on what is considered *normal* at your company.

When the board sits down, do members ask, "What are we

doing to improve safety next month?" Or just, "Are we in compliance with government safety standards?"

When the road crew gathers, does the supervisor say, "Let's do the safety checklist?" Or just, "Be safe out there, guys."

Does a worker turn to another and say, "Hey, don't forget to put on those gloves?" Or do they merely say, "I don't wear gloves, but maybe it's a good idea."

With careful observation, you can characterize your company as it moves up the rungs from "vulnerable" to "reactive," "compliant," "proactive" and finally, "resilient."

THE SAFETY MATURITY LADDER

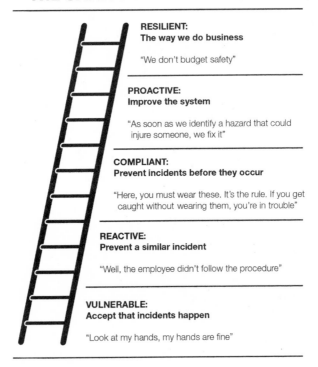

RESILIENT:
The way we do business

"We don't budget safety"

PROACTIVE:
Improve the system

"As soon as we identify a hazard that could injure someone, we fix it"

COMPLIANT:
Prevent incidents before they occur

"Here, you must wear these. It's the rule. If you get caught without wearing them, you're in trouble"

REACTIVE:
Prevent a similar incident

"Well, the employee didn't follow the procedure"

VULNERABLE:
Accept that incidents happen

"Look at my hands, my hands are fine"

At the *vulnerable* stage, a company simply accepts that accidents will happen. Plenty of companies go for decades without moving beyond this rung on the ladder.

Next up is *reactive,* where the company recognizes that *repetitions* of common injuries should be prevented. Still, there's no true hazard assessment looking forward to different kinds of injuries.

From there, a company may get to *compliant,* which is not about government regulations, but about systems and protocols being put in place and enforced—with some kind of real hazard assessment going on. The company knows where the hazards are arising, and when work complies with company safety policies.

Getting to a Systems Approach

The next rung on the ladder represents the largest, most profound step. Movement to the *proactive* rung means that a company or a site, through its culture and methods, embraces a *systems* approach to increasing safety over time. Everyone, top to bottom, *cares,* and takes forward, proactive action based on systematic, proactive hazard assessments. If a machine suddenly starts acting weird and it is deemed unsafe, a *compliant* company will fix it and bring the system back into compliance with its standards. In a *proactive* culture, management will be looking at all the machines and asking, "How can we make the baseline safer?"

Finally, if a company achieves its goals of compliance and proactivity, it can eventually become a truly *resilient* company, having fully integrated safety management into its operations. Everyone, top to bottom, feels *ownership* of the safety issue.

Where is your company on this scale? How can you get to the next step, and the step after? What would it take?

CHAPTER FIVE

THE INFRASTRUCTURE OF HAND SAFETY

You see the big picture on hand safety. You have some clues on psychology. Management and workers are onboard. Now, what specific *infrastructure* changes will save hands at your worksites?

Maybe you're familiar with the standard "hierarchy of safety controls." Everyone seems to know about this way of thinking about protections, but it's often forgotten in day-to-day safety conversations. I want to burn it into your brain.

HIERARCHY OF CONTROLS

MOST EFFECTIVE

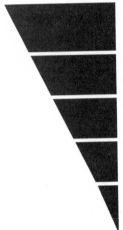

ELIMINATION
Physically remove the hazard

SUBSTITUTION
Replace the hazard

ENGINEERING CONTROLS
Isolate people from the hazard

ADMINISTRATIVE CONTROLS
Change the way people work

PPE
Protect the worker with personal protective equipment

LEAST EFFECTIVE

A logical and rigorous approach to hand safety will *always* start from top to bottom of the hierarchy, as options are explored. The point is to take the *most effective* actions you can to reduce or eliminate injuries, and not automatically skip down to the easier, less-effective solutions lower down—until you are absolutely certain higher-level actions cannot be achieved. That's why the hierarchy is pictured as an upside-down triangle.

I say this even though I am a glove guy, and gloves are, at least theoretically, right at the bottom of the stack.

TWO POINTS TO KEEP IN MIND

Before heading into any discussion of where to make changes, of course, you need to do a genuine *hazard assessment* using the guidelines in chapter nine of this book. Otherwise you are certain to make bad prioritization decisions.

Next, remember that multiple levels of the hierarchy are usually required *simultaneously*. The levels may also need to be implemented in phases, maybe from the bottom up, depending on logistical realities in your company.

Keeping those two points in mind, let's look at the hierarchy in some detail.

WALKING DOWN THE HIERARCHY
ELIMINATION

When you identify a hazard, force yourself to first ask if that hazard can somehow be completely *eliminated*. Seems obvious, right? But it's surprising how often people take a hazard for granted, as in "that's just the way it is."

At my company, we mold gloves on forms. For years, people were at risk of getting carpal tunnel syndrome from the repetitive task of removing gloves from those forms. When we finally thought the problem fully through, we realized we could completely eliminate the carpal risk by adding a compressor that automatically inflates the gloves and pops them right off the form when they're baked. Bingo.

At U.S. Steel, safety experts have for years looked for ways to eliminate the many pinch-point dangers in steel manufacture. Part of their strategy has been to actively design custom "no-touch tools" to eliminate pinch-point hand injury risk from many tasks.[89]

A new tool? A completely different approach? How could a hazard be completely eliminated?

SUBSTITUTION

Second down the hierarchy is *substitution*. If workers have to handle toxic chemicals, they should certainly wear the right chemical-resistant gloves—but could less toxic chemicals be found to do the same job?

If workers are using knives, would retractable box cutters work just as well, reducing the chance of a cut?

If workers have to crimp metal parts, could better, powered crimpers reduce hand muscle strain?

Could a substitution reduce, if not eliminate the risk?

ENGINEERING CONTROLS

Third down the hierarchy are *engineering controls* which basically *isolate people from a hazard*. This includes all manner of safety guards that attempt to keep fingers away from moving gears, blades, grinders, and belts.

Engineering controls can be even more aggressive. If you have a highly hazardous machine, can it be caged and locked out so that only properly trained workers have access? Can the machine be entirely redesigned to make it less dangerous to hands? Could you add an emergency stop switch linked to an electric eye? A trigger grip that has to be held to keep the machine running so it stops the instant the worker lets go? Special handles on boxes to protect fingers?

ADMINISTRATIVE CONTROLS

Okay, suppose you've thought through elimination, substitution, or an engineering redesign to better protect hands. Fourth down the list come *administrative controls.*

This is a big, broad category which can include, for example, redesigning the job instead of the equipment. Can you rotate people into positions on a line to avoid carpal tunnel issues? Can you change the way they reach for parts? The order in which they do the work? Give more breaks to improve concentration?

Administrative controls can also include highly specific warning signs (see later in this chapter), training programs (see chapter eight), emergency wash stations for chemical exposure, safety checklists, supervisory oversight, safety inspections—a long list of possibilities.

It's wrong to think of administrative controls only as a fallback. Why? Because no matter what other controls you put in place, they can never be fully "automatic;" you will always need administrative controls in a hazardous workplace.

FINALLY, WE GET TO PPE

At the bottom of the hierarchy comes *PPE,* or personal protective equipment. Why are things like gloves, sleeves, hard hats, aprons, and seat belts at the bottom of the list? Shouldn't people always wear PPE when doing hazardous work? Well, yes and no. PPE cannot protect against many kinds of hazards, and ultimately, it's the last resort, the final line of protection against a cut, a burn, a chemical exposure, an impact, vibration, a germ exposure, a crash, or you name it.

PPE is the final shield when all other shields have failed.

Unfortunately, it's all too easy to forget that PPE lies at the bottom of the hierarchy. Getting people to wear gloves must never prevent you from exploring all the upper levels of safety actions. Far too often, managers *start* by thinking, "we need better gloves," instead of "how can we eliminate this hazard altogether?"

That said, it's important to remember something else about PPE: Ultimately, you can have all the other levels of the safety hierarchy going, and still miss a critical element. In fact, given the unpredictability of the universe, you will *always* miss a critical element. When the unexpected happens, a glove might be the very thing that saves a worker's hand—and often does.

Indeed, people may need to wear gloves just as a backup when other systems fail.

Paired with Administrative Controls

In any case, remember that like the other levels of the hierarchy, *PPE must always be paired with administrative controls.* Gloves must be mandatory for certain tasks, the right gloves must be provided, they have to be at the right place at the right time, they must be mandated, and they must actually be used. All those are administrative issues.

Like other controls, PPE is *not passive protection*, it is actively deployed for safety.

For a manager, active PPE admin might mean putting up a pegboard with gloves beneath signs for specific tasks. It might mean arranging for a big barrel of gloves in the elevator to the top of the skyscraper construction, ready every single day. It certainly means not assuming workers will buy, bring, and use their own gloves.

JUST BUILD A BOX

Here's a great example of thinking with and without the safety hierarchy.

One of our territory managers visited a paper mill where workers had to carry long, heavy, sharp blades weighing maybe fifty pounds, about 500 feet from the roll-cutting machine to the sharpener several times a day. The manager told our territory manager he needed to find some "super cut-resistant gloves" to protect the workers as they made these journeys. When our TM and the manager went down to visit the mill floor together, it turned out that indeed, a worker had just been injured—but the guy had stabbed himself in the stomach carrying a blade. He'd slipped, and the blade had ripped through his shirt, where he had to have stitches along his belly.

"Um, instead of buying new gloves," offered our rep, "why not build custom wooden boxes to carry around these blades? It'll cost you maybe ten dollars a box to build them. You put the box in a cart and roll it across the factory. You'll save maybe $50,000 a year on fancy gloves, and you won't have the problem at all."

Why were this manager's employees walking around all day carrying huge blades against their bellies? Because the manager had failed to look for an elimination or engineering solution before dropping down to the level of PPE. He'd ignored the hierarchy in his thinking.

Where are you failing to look at a hand injury problem in the larger context of the safety hierarchy?

Overcoming PPE Noncompliance

A big problem with all PPE, and especially with gloves, is noncompliance. Since gloves are an especially personal kind of equipment, workers think they are optional equipment. Sure, you provided the gloves—but are they going to be used?

In addition, gloves are less conspicuous than PPE like helmets, vests, or masks, so others often don't automatically notice if a worker is wearing gloves, and may consider glove-wearing optional, in a different way than say, a construction helmet.

The bottom line? Every minute of every day a worker must make a *decision* on whether to pull on their gloves, pull them off to do delicate work, or lay them aside because their hands are getting hot.

At my company, we've done a systematic analysis of the worker's decision tree. It's surprisingly complex.

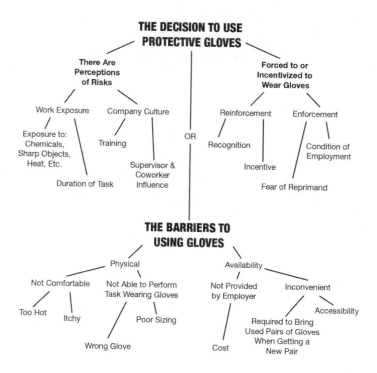

Where can you use this decision tree to open the eyes of managers and workers, and to increase compliance with glove-wearing?

TWO MORE NOTES ON THE HIERARCHY OF SAFETY

Before we leave the famous, vital, and never-to-be-ignored hierarchy of safety, I just want to add two more personal notes. You might even call them amendments.

ALL AVAILABLE MEANS

Useful as the hierarchy may be, it may falsely give the impression that you should only focus on the highest level possible, while ignoring other levels. I already said you should assume you will need multiple levels of the hierarchy simultaneously—but let me go further now and point out that when you are trying to prevent accidents to human beings, you are going to use all available means. You're going to use *all* levels of the hierarchy that you can.

If I were in charge of safety at, say, a skyscraper construction site, I would be ashamed if an accident occurred because I had not used all available means at my disposal.

NO BROKEN WINDOWS

My second note may sound trivial, but it is not. The hierarchy of safety doesn't just live within the emotional culture of a company, it lives within the physical culture of a company.

So housekeeping matters. A lot.

Back in the 1990s the crime rate in New York City was brought down precipitously by what was known as the "broken window theory." Policies based on this theory led the police and the courts to crack down on even the most trivial of offenses: breaking a window, putting graffiti on a bus, jaywalking. Streets were cleaned up. Garbage was collected.[90]

The psychological effect of living in a cleaner city where people cared about small crimes led to huge improvements in the larger issues of human behavior. Major crimes dropped when minor crimes were prosecuted.

I absolutely think you cannot implement any safety hierarchy in a physical environment which includes heaps of trash, unclean floors, or yes, broken windows. A sense of order must prevail before elimination, substitution, engineering, administration, or PPE can do their work.

At one shipyard,[91] the safety manager figured that 50 percent of accidents were linked in some way to untidy conditions—bits of metal left lying around, scattered tools, unclean tools, you name it. This safety manager promised headquarters that if house-keeping were improved, injuries could be reduced by around 25 percent. In reality, after a rigorous housekeeping initiative, injuries dropped by an astounding 70 percent—which meant that injuries of all kinds were being reduced. Why? Everyone, top to bottom, was acting in a safer manner because they were acting in a clean, controlled environment.

How can you make sure that your safety policies exist within an overall sense of orderliness in the work environment?

KEY ISSUES FOR HAND GUARDS AND OTHER ENGINEERING SOLUTIONS

It's beyond the scope of this book to talk about specific engineering solutions, like hand guards for particular kinds of equipment. But here are key points to keep in mind when engineering *any* solution:

1. Don't assume that the OEM (original equipment manufacturer) guard on a machine is good enough. Many companies rightly consider OEM safety equipment only the starting point.

2. An actual, day-to-day operator of the machine should be involved in safety guard design. Incredibly obvious as this may seem, actual operators are often left out of the design conversation. On the other hand, experts who are not oper-

ators of the machine should also be involved—because they will look with fresh eyes, and see things the operator, through over-familiarity, may not. *By using both operators and non-operator design experts, you can go a long way in overcoming the cognitive biases we discussed in chapter three.*

3. In general, it's wrong to think about safety guards as "passive" protection. It must be absolutely clear to workers why a guard was put in place on a machine. They must then *consciously and actively* use and maintain that guard.

4. Workers often disable safety guards because they are in the way and slow down the task. Don't just tell them to use a machine "only with a guard device" without explaining (or better yet, demonstrating) what happens without that device. In training, emphasize that disabling guards is a substantial and ever-present risk which causes many hand accidents. *Indeed, people can sometimes be criminally prosecuted for disabling safety guards.*[92]

5. As an engineering solution, see if a redesign could include a way of disabling the machine when the safety guard is removed.

MAKING LOCKOUT/TAGOUT A PRIORITY

Many hand injuries occur because a machine is started up unexpectedly, particularly during a maintenance cycle. Plenty of additional injuries occur because dangerous machinery, tools, or electrical circuits are accessed by people who should not have access at all.

Horror stories are common. Someone is working under a conveyor belt when someone else flips the on switch...you get the idea.

A safety manager needs to implement rigorous systems of

locking out dangerous machinery when not in use, or at least tagging it with a "Do Not Start—Maintenance Underway" sign when appropriate.

Lockout/tagout is often a case of looking forward to anticipate a type of injury which has never occurred before. Indeed, workers may be so accustomed to using a particular piece of machinery that they do not think about the unintended results of turning it on at the wrong time, or letting the untrained try to use it.

Lockout/tagout is also a clear situation in which policy, training, and infrastructure must be carefully coordinated.

1. Does a supervisor have to sign out the equipment or provide a key?
2. Are workers, including workers with poor local language skills, looking for the big orange tags that indicate someone is working on this equipment, so stay clear? Or are there so many signs in the environment that they ignore lockout tags?
3. What system is in place to ensure that lockout/tagout happens every single time it is needed?

A LOCKOUT/TAGOUT HORROR STORY

The largest fine for a safety violation ever levied in California came from an incident in 2012 when a worker named José Melena, aged sixty-two, was burned alive while cleaning out a thirty-five-foot oven at a Bumble Bee tuna canning factory. Because two of his coworkers failed to lock and tag the oven for the cleaning, other workers loaded six tons of tuna into the oven, unknowingly trapping Melena. Then the oven was turned on. Later, the workers said they thought Melena was in the restroom at the time. His remains were found two hours later.

Bumble Bee was fined over $6 million. Some $1.5 million went to Melena's family as compensation. The two coworkers who failed to lockout/tagout the oven were criminally charged. Bumble Bee was also forced to install new safety equipment and add considerable training for their managers and workers.[93]

KEY ISSUES IN DESIGNING SIGNS

Signage can make a huge difference in hand safety but only the right signage. All signs are definitely not equal, and far too little thought is usually given to actual design.

Look around your facility. Is there a sign that reads "Warning High Voltage?" It's useless. How does someone avoid the high voltage? What gloves should they wear, exactly, when entering the electrical room? Who is allowed in?

Here are some golden rules of good safety sign design:

1. In the United States, OSHA has specific design standards, including colors, for safety signs. You can easily download the latest information on these standards—which are highly recommended, even if you are not in the US.[94]

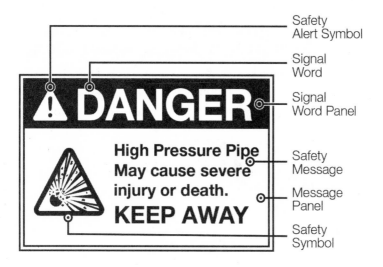

2. Signs need to be big and bold enough to be noticed. Too often, signs are overly subtle.

3. Signs must be placed at eye height, not way up near the ceiling or by the floor. They must be unmistakably close to the hazard. Too often, signs are placed at random heights, where they go unnoticed. Machines get moved, but the signs don't go with them.

4. Safety sign design and coloring should be consistent throughout a facility. Signs in a different design may not be noticed. Simple solution: follow the OSHA standard.

5. Signs must contain the right level of information for someone to: a) fully understand the risk; and b) actually *take the right steps* to stay safe. A sign without both of these requirements will be completely ineffective. If you post a sign saying, "Use Caution When Operating Cutting Machine" you have wasted your time. Think about it: such a sign fulfills neither requirement.

In Florida, you often see signs warning about alligators. But the effective signs give you more information than just "Beware of Alligators." They say things like, "Avoid alligator attacks by staying away from tall grass and water."[95] Now I know that alligators may attack, and I know how to avoid them. Here's an example provided by Clarion Safety Systems, which supplied new signs to the Disney Resort in Florida, after a tragedy.

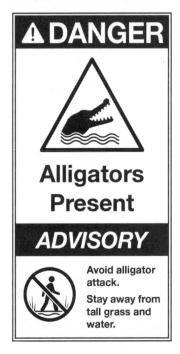

In the below example, the top sign makes an attempt to get past a mere "Caution" warning, but it does not give enough information to clearly understand the danger and avoid it. What can get crushed? And how? By adding the explanatory image, the sign becomes useful.

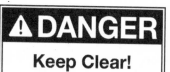
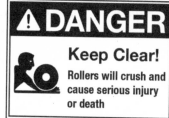

Source: GraphicProducts.com, used with permission. Thanks to Joel Bradbury.

6. Photos or pictograms like that on the second sign above can convey information much more quickly and with a higher impact than words. The right images can also overcome language barriers. But when you use pictograms, always add explanatory words, particularly to tell workers how to avoid the dangers. *Make pictograms plus words your default choice for all signage.*

Here are some more examples of bad, old-fashioned signage vs. modern effective signage, again from Clarion.

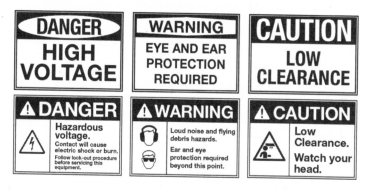

1. These examples are only in English, but never assume that adding a pictogram makes up for posting a sign only in English (or the primary local language). If you have a multilingual workforce, you must *also translate* any text to ensure understanding.

2. Signs need to state that certain actions are *mandatory*. Don't say, "Wear gloves when handling metal parts." Say, "Level 3 cut-resistant gloves are mandatory when handling metal parts." Don't say, "Lock out the electrical room when not in use," say "Lockout of electrical room is mandatory when not in use."

3. As we said in chapter two, mistake #5, signs must never imply that people are stupid for not wearing gloves or taking other safety actions. Never say, "Don't be stupid, wear your gloves." This is terrible for morale.

4. Never joke on a safety sign. It is disrespectful to those in danger and creates a separation between management and workers.

5. As we discussed in chapter three, in the section on the uses of fear, it is my opinion that you should never put up a sign showing a horrible injury next to a machine or elsewhere. Over time, this causes denial and deliberate avoidance of looking at the sign, not safety, and is demoralizing. Such images may be used in training, with caution, as we discuss in chapter eight, but not on signs.

6. Positive role model signs work. Instead of a picture of somebody's fingers that got cut off, you could have a picture of a smiling guy wearing the right gloves, and say, "Joe has an 80 percent lower chance of a hand injury because he's wearing level 5 cut-resistant gloves." Below, I've included a huge sign placed in a factory in Bogota showing a lifesize photo of a worker correctly suited up. This offers great positive reinforcement.

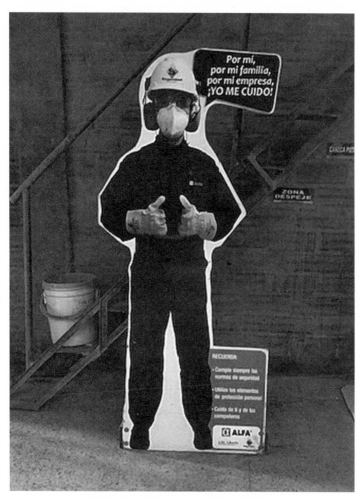

7. Signs should be rotated out and replaced from time to time: people just stop noticing signs they see every day. *Establish a regular replacement schedule.*

PUTTING IT ALL TOGETHER

Angela Lambert and Derek Eversdyke of Clarion link the hierarchy of safety controls to good, modern signage, and echo my emphasis on multiple layers of protection:

"The safety profession has embraced the concept of 'hierarchy of controls' for many years—it's not new. But what is interesting is that many of the safety professionals who use the hierarchy of controls believe the steps described in a typical chart are choices to be used in an 'either/or' kind of way, not in a layered 'both/and' approach. But the latter approach defines how the hierarchy of controls is meant to be evaluated and used as a means to control risk.

"For example, a machine has moving parts that create an entanglement hazard. The hazard cannot be eliminated, so the equipment manufacturer installed a guard on the machine (let's assume the guard is removable to clear jams and maintain the equipment). The manufacturer has also placed a warning label on the guard that says, 'Entanglement hazard. Do not operate with guard removed. Lockout/tagout before servicing.' The equipment manufacturer has done three things related to the hierarchy of controls to mitigate this risk associated with their machine:

- Installed a guard.
- Warned about the hazard.
- Instructed how to avoid the hazard.

"Now let's take this same example and explore it from the perspective of the safety professional looking to mitigate the risk of entanglement in the same machine in their workplace. They can do the following:

- Put in place a procedure that inspects equipment on each shift to make sure the machine's guards are in place.
- Put in place a procedure that inspects the machine monthly to make sure its warning labels are intact and legible.

- Implement safety training for all machine operators and maintenance personnel who could possibly interact with this machine's entanglement hazard to instruct them on how to safely clear jams and service the equipment.
- Install a facility safety sign that instructs people on how to safely lockout/tagout the equipment as a means to reinforce the safety training that has taken place. Additional signage could be installed that communicates the need to wear proper PPE when operating or in the vicinity of the machine (e.g., eye protection, hearing protection, wearing or not wearing gloves, no loose clothing/jewelry/long hair, etc.).

"With best practice labels on the machinery and complimentary warnings within the facility, the worker is given a consistent system of warnings that can help them to avoid injuries to hands, fingers and other body parts while using the machine."[96]

I would just add that the safety professional should go a little further and carefully examine the OEM guards to see if they could be improved.

Now you're talking *infrastructure*.

CHAPTER SIX

FOR WANT OF A (PROPER) GLOVE

Choosing a glove may seem like a small decision, but if the work you do endangers hands, this "small decision" will have a huge impact. I guarantee it. Maybe you've heard this old proverb, passed down through the centuries:

> *For want of a nail the shoe was lost*
> *For want of a shoe the horse was lost*
> *For want of a horse the rider was lost*
> *For want of a rider the message was lost*
> *For want of a message the battle was lost*
> *For want of a battle the kingdom was lost*
> *And all for the want of a horseshoe nail*

Let me kick off this chapter with an updated version for the industrial age:

> *For want of a glove, a finger was lost*
> *For want of a finger, a worker was lost*

For want of a worker, the schedule was lost
For want of a schedule, a customer was lost
For want of a customer, the year was lost
For want of a year, the company was lost
All for the want of a proper glove

I'm no poet, but you get the idea. I have spent my entire life in gloves. I grew up in Acton, Canada, where the smell of the leather tanneries hung in the air day and night. I started helping my father make and sell gloves when I was eight. After I got a degree in chemistry, I was sent to study at the Reutlingen leather school in Germany, which you might call the "Hogwarts of leather making." I continue to work in the family business, which has grown into one of North America's biggest glove suppliers.

So believe me when I say that the very most important word in my reworking of the old proverb comes in the last line, and it's the word "proper."

SUMMARIZING THE PROBLEM IN A SINGLE LINE

This chapter is about how to choose the *proper* glove to protect your workers: on factory floors, up on skyscraper skeletons, out on deepwater rigs, laying asphalt along roadbeds, handling contaminated sharps down in hospital labs.

The chapter is not a comprehensive look at glove options—that would take another whole book, which would have to be reissued every few months, because new designs and materials appear regularly. If you are seriously in need of gloves, you will need to sit down with a knowledgeable representative of a major glove manufacturer to choose the proper pair for the exact tasks your workers perform. In fact, you need an ongoing relationship, not a one-off fling.

Nevertheless, in this chapter I can up your game with a few choice pieces of advice. In fact, I can summarize a lifetime of experience into a single line:

> The proper glove is the one that meets the minimum requirements, and that people will actually wear.

Each word in that line is important:

I say "minimum," because with gloves, you don't want overkill. They must not be too bulky, too expensive, or too overdesigned for the work, because they won't get used.

By "requirements," I don't just mean government standards. I mean clearly understanding what's actually needed in terms of protection, grip, dexterity, comfort, etc., top and bottom— *for that very particular task.* That means close study, talking to workers, trying out different options.

When I say "and that people will actually wear," I'm acknowledging that people often refuse to wear gloves, or they remove their gloves at the worst possible moment. A Liberty Mutual study found that about 70 percent of hand injuries happen because people aren't wearing gloves when they should have.[97] *Often enough, they weren't wearing their gloves because they literally couldn't do their jobs with the gloves on.*

By "people," I mean the actual workers, on the job, in the moment, when they go through that decision process to wear or not wear their gloves that I outlined in the last chapter. By "people," I definitely don't mean the purchasing manager or the supervisor or the safety trainer, even though all those others will help select the gloves.

By "actually wear," I mean you have to seriously consider comfort, sweatiness, dexterity, hot and cold, ugliness and style—because again, *gloves provide absolutely no protection if they are not worn.*

My company makes over 1,000 different kinds of work gloves because that's how many it takes to fit all the kinds of work and safety minimums of our customers, along with all the kinds of comfort and style needed to fulfill that otherwise simple dictum.

MOST COMMON REASONS EMPLOYEES DO NOT WEAR GLOVES

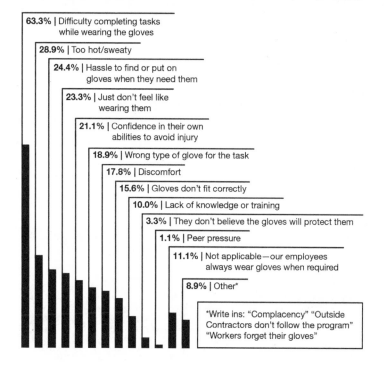

63.3% | Difficulty completing tasks while wearing the gloves

28.9% | Too hot/sweaty

24.4% | Hassle to find or put on gloves when they need them

23.3% | Just don't feel like wearing them

21.1% | Confidence in their own abilities to avoid injury

18.9% | Wrong type of glove for the task

17.8% | Discomfort

15.6% | Gloves don't fit correctly

10.0% | Lack of knowledge or training

3.3% | They don't believe the gloves will protect them

1.1% | Peer pressure

11.1% | Not applicable—our employees always wear gloves when required

8.9% | Other*

*Write ins: "Complacency" "Outside Contractors don't follow the program" "Workers forget their gloves"

THE NEW STUFF IS AMAZINGLY BETTER

I grew up working with leather. I love leather gloves. Leather is still great for some kinds of work, but I also need to say up front that a pure leather glove is now mostly obsolete for most tasks. It's just animal skin, and no matter how great it feels, leather gets cut like animal skin, offers little impact resistance, and it's nearly as porous as human skin to dangerous chemicals.

In general, you will find synthetic gloves available now that offer far higher levels of protection along with incredible dexterity and comfort. You can use them while tying your shoes, working your iPhone, you name it. Kevlar and Dyneema, for example, are true miracle fibers—and in a few years, I'm sure other materials will emerge. Whatever gloves you have been using, you need to keep trying out the new stuff, because the new stuff rocks.

At my company, we invest heavily in R&D. The availability and quality of modern materials pushes us forward every day. Don't let your company get left behind, ever. At the very least, don't fall for the tired myth that leather is somehow always best, and other choices are cheap imitations.

You can read some more specifics about leather in Appendix 1C.

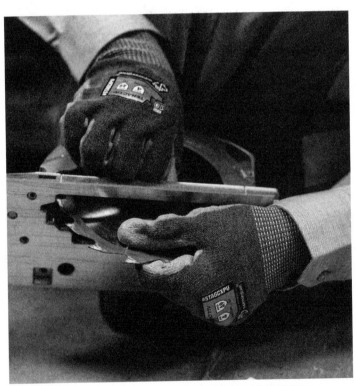

New materials can provide both dexterity and cut resistance at the same time.

FASHION MATTERS

If you think it's ridiculous to bring up fashion in a work glove, you are dead wrong. When you're talking about getting men or women to wear their gloves regularly, you'd better believe it matters how the gloves look. Here's a simple rule:

Gloves should play into machismo, not against it.

When you're fighting a macho attitude among men (and women) that says, "I'm too tough to wear gloves," it helps to give them gloves that make them look *more* tough. Why not hand them work gloves that look like NASCAR driving gloves or dirt bike sporting gloves? Pulling on those puppies might just feel great.

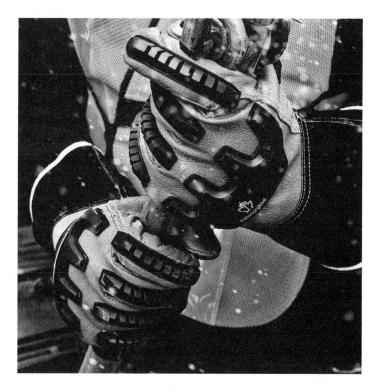

Once our folks were working with a company in Columbus, Ohio, where everyone was crazy for Ohio State. We gave them the choice of two or three gloves and they eagerly chose the red model just because it echoed the look of Ohio State. Maybe this glove was not the absolute best selection in terms of the task, but fine: glove compliance shot way up.

Are you thinking of buying fluorescent orange gloves so people don't lose them? Think twice.

On the flip side, I do have to mention that we've had purchasing managers turn down our very cool-looking camouflage gloves because they thought they looked *too* good, and the employees would be taking them home a little too often. And of course, ultimately safety does have to outweigh fashion. Go back to my one-liner about "minimum requirements." Camo styling doesn't make a work glove any safer.

HOW NOT TO CHOOSE A GLOVE

The most frustrating part of my job comes when the purchaser has no interest in my experience, the availability of modern materials, or the fine balance between protection, comfort, cost, launderability, and fashion. Far too many times I've sat with a purchasing agent at a large company, started a conversation about running worker trials with different models and materials, and had the agent shut me down by saying:

> We've been using this same kind of glove for twenty years. I just want to know if you can give me a better price.

Normally I can't say what I'm thinking, so I'll say it here:

Listen friend, if you've been using the same gloves for twenty years, you are doing a profound disservice to your workers. Why? Because gloves have improved, tasks have undoubtedly changed, and I know for a fact that you could do a better job protecting your people's hands.

I realize it's not just a hassle, it's psychologically tough to change gloves. It's like changing a favorite brand of jeans—on 100 or 200 people. But sorry, that's no excuse for not improving your safety. Would you use the same cell phone you used twenty years ago? Gloves have improved just as much.

GIVING LOW-PAID WORKERS CRAPPIER GLOVES THAN HIGHLY PAID WORKERS

Here's another sad truth about glove choice.

Too often, I see great gloves provided to highly paid workers; with cheap or no PPE given to low-paid workers, despite the fact that the lower-paid workers are likely doing more hazardous work.

Yup, that's a reality.

In the oil and gas industry, where a drill operator may earn US $80 an hour, the company will want to keep the operator happy, and no one seems to mind paying $30 for a pair of gloves with full impact and cut-resistance.

In residential construction, equally dangerous to hands, I too often see worn-out gloves with little or no cut resistance. Or worse, no gloves at all provided by management.

The food processing industry suffers from an extremely high hand injury rate, but management tends to be highly cost conscious and the hourly wage for workers is very low. Again, when I visit food processing plants, I often see completely inadequate gloves.

I try to explain to every client in every industry that good gloves actually save money in the long run. As we discussed in chapter four, the ROI is actually pretty obvious: A glove may cost twice as much, but it may last four times longer, stand up to laundering, and most importantly, prevent lost time to injuries, improve morale—and much more.[98] Need I add that providing the appropriate glove for each task is also just *the right thing to do*—regardless of a worker's annual compensation package?

Are you unconsciously aligning glove quality with wage rates?

OTHER WAYS NOT TO CHOOSE A GLOVE

Picking a glove without a hazard assessment. Sure, worker hands need to be protected against cuts and abrasions. But do they also face a good chance of an impact? Occasional chemical exposure? Even if no such injuries have yet occurred, you need to find out if they could. Far too often, gloves are chosen based only on *past* injuries, without trying to *anticipate* dangers. Even more often, a purchasing manager opens a catalog, points, and says, "These should be fine."

Picking a glove without running sample trials with actual workers. You absolutely need worker feedback, and actual workers need to tell you that yes, these gloves can be used when performing this task, or no, they're too clumsy. Actual workers need to say, "I guess these gloves are comfortable enough—so yeah, these gloves will get worn." Later in this chapter, I'll talk about how to run these trials.

Letting workers choose their own gloves, with no oversight. I've walked into facilities where I've seen upwards of 100 or 200 different kinds of gloves being worn. I'll turn to the safety manager and say, "What's going on? You probably need ten different kinds of gloves, not a hundred, right?" And the reply comes, "Well, Jack likes this brand, and Jill likes that brand, so we let everyone choose their own. We give them a catalog, and they just specify what they want, and we order it."

I carefully explain that not only does this cause a staggeringly unnecessary expense, but individual workers simply do not have the expertise to each choose their own glove. They don't know the options, they don't know all the issues, and they won't put in the necessary time for the decision.

Worker input, yes. Worker free-for-all, no.

MILLENNIALS GIVE E-COMMERCE TOO MUCH LOVE

One problem with letting workers randomly choose their own gloves is the tendency of millennials to assume that one-off, online glove prices are somehow great prices. Plenty of times, younger workers will go to Amazon and pay three times the price for a pair of gloves that the company could get far more cheaply in bulk through their purchasing department.

For example, Canadian Rail told me they once negotiated a price of CN $5/pair for a certain type of glove. But their younger workers were too impatient to deal with their purchasing department, so even after the deal, these workers were buying the identical gloves on Amazon for $15/pair—on the company account.

Next day delivery? Sure. Economy and consistency? Not so much.

Relying on a distributor instead of talking directly to experts at a glove company. We once ran a secret shopper test in which we called up some major distributors and said, "Hey, we're a metal-stamping company with 300 employees. We just had a serious hand injury and we're using X kind of glove—what would you recommend?" The responses were shocking. Usually distributors asked us exactly what kind of glove we were using, then said, "Great, I've got that glove, but I can give it to you for a little less than you're paying." Seriously? The same gloves in which our people got injured, but lower quality? No advice on upgrading for safety? Distributors, of course, sell everything from nuts and bolts to compressors and forklift parts. It's not surprising they can't always offer expert opinions on gloves. If you are a concern of any size, a serious glove company should be willing to come assess your needs, run trials, and get you the right stuff.

Ignoring questions like laundering and expected usable life. If you have upwards of fifty employees, these questions get expensive, fast. Can or can't the gloves be washed? How long will they last? I discuss laundering in detail later in this chapter.

Focusing on covering your ass instead of your workers' safety. If your primary question is, "Will this glove keep OSHA off our back and prevent us from getting sued?" you are going down the wrong path. Most likely result? You will buy gloves that are bulky and overprotective—hence they won't get worn. When someone loses a finger you might not get sued for failure to provide adequate PPE, but if you'd bought the right kind of glove, the guy might have actually been wearing his gloves and his finger may not have been hurt at all.

Here's one of the most common questions I get from purchasing managers: "What do you have that protects against basically everything?"

The answer? "The total glove exists, but you don't want it. We have gloves that allow you to hold something that's 1,000 degrees Fahrenheit, but no one can wear it to hold a nail and hammer it in." If you add puncture resistance, you are adding bulk. If you make a glove waterproof you are not just adding bulk, but discomfort. The trade-offs are real, and the trade-offs require expert advice, trials, and worker feedback, not CYA.

Thinking "one person, one pair of gloves." A construction worker might spend the early morning handling a jackhammer requiring vibration-protective gloves. By 10 a.m., she might be handling a hazardous chemical like a tar or glue. Later, she might pick up a smoothing rasp requiring an entirely different kind of protection. Ideally, that worker would switch gloves for each task—with the glove associated to the task, not the worker. Too often, however, both workers and supervisors think, "That's the glove for Jane," instead of, "That's the glove for jackhammering." *The right prescription is "one task, one pair of gloves."* The more specific the better.

GLOVES AND PURCHASING MANAGERS

This book includes a good deal of frustration with purchasing managers. But let's be clear: if you are a safety manager, you need to work closely with your purchasing manager when you go looking for gloves, and you have to support your purchasing manager's need to control costs.

Purchasing managers rarely have much expertise in either the specific work being performed or in the different kinds of PPE. Hard hats, reflective vests, aprons, and safety goggles aren't all that specialized—but gloves are a deep and complex topic in which major trade-offs in cost, quality, protection, fashion, launderability, dexterity, comfort, and all the rest must be considered.

If you are a safety manager, it's you who will do the homework on hazard assessments. It's you who will work with the representative of a major glove company to run worker trials and consider all the options. But it will also be you who may have to convince the purchasing manager to go from a two-dollar glove to a twenty-dollar glove. That will take careful research and case building.

If you are a purchasing manager, you have to recognize that buying gloves for 1,000 people is not like buying coffee cups for 1,000 people. It's not hard to develop expertise in buying coffee cups, but gloves are highly specialized, and people's lives depend on them. You shouldn't go it alone, and you don't have to—glove manufacturers will do the research for you, and provide the supporting ROI information, too.

I could write a horror movie featuring a PM my company has dealt with at a certain auto parts manufacturer. The workers there are machining metal, handling greased parts, fitting heavy bolts, driving rivets. Year after year, this PM buys his workers cheap cotton gloves, literally the kind designed for light gardening that cost maybe US $0.25 a pair in bulk. Year after year, our reps show up to explain how better gloves are needed in this factory and please, *please* let us do an assessment. But year after year, this PM just stares us down and says: "All I want is to see a lower price on the same gloves." In the horror movie, the camera would switch right from his steely stare to the factory floor, where we'd see people getting fingers crushed, cut, and soaked in carcinogenic lubricants.[99]

Don't be that PM. And if you *are* that PM, I pray you are reading this book.

THE RIGHT WAY TO BUY GLOVES

The right way to buy gloves follows a rigorous plan:

1. Do a hazard assessment *per task,* or better yet, do an assessment in tandem with a reputable glove company. They'll probably do it for free. See chapter seven on how to do a hazard assessment right.
2. Identify the requirements for each kind of glove, per task. You can use the next section for a checklist of possible requirements. As you make your list, you may realize that you need ten or more different kinds of gloves in your facility. I've seen factories that needed twenty different kinds of gloves to cover all their different kinds of tasks. One reason you need different gloves for different tasks is that you must not overprotect: overly bulky, hot, or uncomfortable gloves will not be worn. *Again: one task, one type of glove.*
3. Ask a glove manufacturer to supply multiple glove samples for each task type requiring different kinds of gloves. Only two or three glove options will be all you need for a trial against each task, plus the incumbent glove. As part

of choosing the gloves for the trial, you need to be up front with your glove company about your criteria for success. You might say, "We want a glove that meets all the requirements we've listed for this task, but lasts 50 percent longer than the incumbent glove, and reduces our costs by 10 percent, overall." *Then let them choose the samples to try out.*

4. Run trials (see the section below) with a selection of actual workers performing the actual tasks and fill out trial evaluation forms. Don't let one worker, one supervisor, or one PM make this decision.

5. Put together the data from trials, compare prices, and negotiate bulk deals on your multiple glove types for multiple tasks. You can find samples of trial data aggregation in Appendix 2.

POSSIBLE GLOVE REQUIREMENTS

When you set out to buy gloves, you need to compile a clear set of requirements to discuss with a manufacturer, based on your hazard assessment. As you compile these requirements, I want you to remember my dictum once again:

The proper glove is the one that meets the minimum requirements, but that people will actually wear.

If you find you need a cut level 2, don't even test out a cut level 5—it will be too bulky. As with Goldilocks, "just right" is just right. You should think through each of the requirements below, and become familiar with any of the specific industry/government standards that apply to your work.

Here's my checklist:

- **Dexterity.** There are standards for dexterity, but really you need to run specific trials to understand the dexterity needs of your workers.
- **Grip.** Also requires specific trials to understand needs, and the gloves may require special coatings. Sheet metal, for example, is usually covered in a metal-handling oil to prevent rust—and you need the exact right glove for the work. If you're making a large sheet of glass, say for the skin of a highrise, you need an extremely good grip, along with cut resistance: if the glass slips, you instinctively tighten your grip, and the glass can cut through you like a blade. "General purpose" gloves will not suffice.
- **Cut resistance.** Modern materials have revolutionized cut resistance. For example, Kevlar, the same material used in bulletproof vests, can be spun into thread and knitted into gloves to provide remarkable cut resistance. If you're wearing the correct glove and a piece of glass slides into your hand, you may not get cut, or if you do get cut, the wound will be far less severe. You should make your choice based on standard ANSI cut levels. You'll find this, and most of the standards on the supporting website at www.rethinkinghandsafety.com. But this one is so important, I'm putting the standard here for you to study.

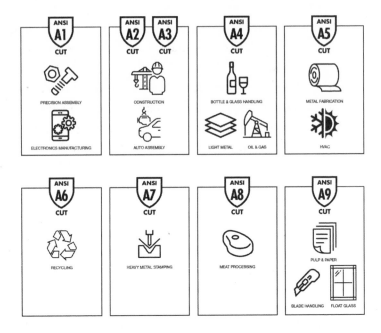

- **Abrasion resistance.** Abrasion injuries are second only to cuts, but abrasion resistance also relates to the overall life of the glove. I have seen manufacturing environments, for example, where even high-quality gloves must be changed out for a new pair four times a day. Note that leather still provides great abrasion resistance, but modern materials are catching up fast. If your work includes substantial abrasion, you will want to run a glove trial long enough to see if the glove holds up over time.
- **Puncture resistance.** When choosing gloves for puncture resistance, you need to know if you are specifically dealing with small objects like needles, or larger objects like broken glass. You will find specific standards for each. Puncture resistance always reduces dexterity and comfort, so difficult choices must be made. See Appendix 1B for more detail.
- **Impact resistance.** These gloves include padding on the top of the hand and the fingers, and evolved out of sporting

gloves like those used for dirt biking. Some industries often expose workers to severe impact dangers, especially from heavy equipment—and over the last few years, impact-resistant gloves have dramatically reduced things like back hand fractures in the oil and gas industry. They are surprisingly comfortable. You will find a link to understanding the latest rating impact resistance standards in Appendix 1F.

- **Heat resistance.** Industry has made huge strides in protecting workers from heat dangers through automation and tool redesign, but in certain applications, gloves remain crucial for handling things like hot cooking oil, welded parts, and molten metals. Heat-resistant gloves have specific temperature ratings, and you need to do careful research on what you require.

- **Vibration resistance.** Vital for workers using pneumatic tools or similar equipment which can cause HAVS, hand-arm vibration syndrome, a serious disability. For tools with high levels of vibration, like a jackhammer, choose a glove with a lot of anti-vibration padding; for smaller tools like a grinder, go with a thinner, more formfitting glove. A glove with too much padding can actually increase forearm strain and increase the likelihood of HAVS. Also full-finger gloves are much better than half-finger versions, as HAVS is most likely to develop in the fingertips. See Appendix 1G for more about these kinds of gloves.

- **Hazardous substances protection.** There's no such thing as "generic hazardous substances protection." If a job includes the handling of chemicals, it's critical for your glove company to know exactly *which* chemicals, so the glove or glove coatings can be exactly right. For example, there's a glove made of polyvinyl alcohol that's resistant to a wide range of quite hazardous chemicals, but it's soluble in water. If it comes in contact with water, it will fall apart quickly.

Importantly, no chemical-resistant glove will keep the bad stuff out forever. You need to know how long a resistant glove can hold out, and when it needs to be thrown away.

- **Microorganism protection.** Disposable gloves used mostly in healthcare applications. Make sure to also consider abrasion resistance, puncture resistance, allergies, powdering, and more.

- **Winter warmth.** Good winter gloves for industrial uses have always presented a challenge—how do you make a glove that's warm, flexible, and cut resistant all at the same time? For how long must it keep a worker's hand warm at say, minus 20 Fahrenheit, before the worker runs back inside? At what point does a bulky glove become a hazard? Any good winter work glove will have multiple layers, manage moisture effectively, and stay warm even at the fingertips. The lining should be wool, polypropylene, or Thinsulate®—never cotton.

- **Length of cuffs or separate sleeves.** Are your worker's arms also in danger from burns, cuts, and abrasions? If you need a cut-resistant glove, it's likely you also need a long cuff or a separate protective sleeve. See a detailed discussion under Appendix 1E.

- **Custom requirements.** Do workers finish up a task by pushing in a pin with the palm of their hand? Maybe you need a glove with a thick pad right at that spot. Do you need extra cut protection along the thumb? Large manufacturers may have what you need, or may custom design a glove—do your homework and *be specific*.

- **Laundering ability.** A question often ignored during a glove selection process, but crucial to long-term value and total cost. I discuss laundering in a section below.

- **Coatings.** An enormous number of specialized coatings are available for work gloves, either for the entire glove or just for the palm and underside of the fingers. These coatings may apply to a variety of needs above, and you definitely need expert help in selecting the right coating. See Appendix 1D for a reference chart for the basics on some current coatings.

- **Comfort and fit.** The question of comfort and fit is vital to all glove types, but comfort requirements may depend greatly on the length of time each glove is worn for a specific task. That makes a real-world trial even more important.

UNDERSTANDING GLOVE LIMITATIONS

I noted above that no chemical-resistant gloves work for all chemicals, and no glove will hold out against *any* toxic substance forever.

Just as there are no chemical-proof gloves, only *chemical-resistant* gloves, there are no cut-proof gloves. If you take a pair of scissors to a level 5 *cut-resistant* glove, you will eventually manage to cut through it.

There are no impact-proof gloves, only *impact-resistant* gloves.

And so on.

Whenever you select gloves, both you and your workers need to understand the real-world limitations of those gloves.

Indeed, in certain situations, gloves may be worse than bare hands. For example, gloves can get caught in rotating machinery like lathes or drill presses, and pull off fingers or whole hands. (There are some glove manufacturers that promote "tear away" gloves. At my company, we advocate against using these as we feel they still increase your odds of getting pulled into rotating equipment versus no gloves. You might be protecting yourself against a cut but increasing your odds of amputating your hand. Not a great risk/reward ratio.)

Gloves can create a danger if chemicals soak through and stay inside the glove. Some people will be allergic to certain materials, like latex. Very tiny parts may make gloves impossible to use. Ill-fitting gloves may create special hazards: for example, gloves that are too big may be grabbed more readily by moving machinery.

You need expert help in understanding these limitations as part of the selection and later training processes.

You also need to remember the hierarchy of safety controls in chapter five: Never forget that gloves, like all personal protective equipment, are only the last line of defense, when all other defenses have failed.

ABOUT LAUNDERING

You may have been surprised to see "launderability" in the requirements' checklist above. You may even have scoffed and said to yourself, "We would never bother washing our gloves—it's impossible." And it's true that most companies will simply throw out even highly expensive, custom gloves when they become overly sweaty or dirty.

I'd like you to reconsider that attitude, if at all practical within your company. It bothers me that more companies don't try to wash gloves. I find it a tremendous waste of money and resources.

If you pay $10 for a pair of gloves, and you manage to launder them just once at a cost of $.50, you've saved $9.50. If you manage to launder and re-use the pair twice, you've saved $19.00. In a company with thousands of employees, that can add up to real money.

The companies with the best records in laundering are in manufacturing, where gloves can be easily collected and returned. Only rarely does a construction concern or an oil and gas company make the attempt, given the difficulty of the logistics—but more should.

I understand you may get pushback from workers who don't want to wear a washed glove, or have some kind of negative reaction to wearing a glove someone else wore; but if a glove is laundered properly, those concerns can be overcome. After all, in a restaurant, everyone takes it for granted that their fork has been used by hundreds of other people, and they're fine with that as long as they believe the fork has been cleaned properly.

I grant you that laundering gloves is not easy. You may harm the gloves in the process, including destroying important coatings. Do the laundering poorly, and workers will waste a lot of time sorting through bins of washed gloves to find a pair that's still in decent condition.

The secret is to use a professional glove laundering company. Such companies exist, and they bring genuine expertise to the laundering process—including protecting the vital properties of the gloves and making sure they feel and smell fresh for employees. I provide a link in Appendix 1H.

UPCOMING TECHNOLOGIES

I've said that it's your responsibility to work with a major glove manufacturer so you stay up-to-date with advances in things like cut-resistance and impact-resistance. But other technologies are beginning to emerge which will revolutionize the whole concept of the glove. Most of these have to do with predictive and sensor technologies.

One recently developed glove can tell you that a worker has been moving their hand in a way likely to cause carpal tunnel injuries. Another kind of glove may warn workers when they get too close to a hazard, or warn them that they have been too long in a hot environment. At my company we're also working on gloves that stay flexible and dexterous until a sudden impact stiffens and hardens them, instantly protecting the hand.

RUNNING GLOVE TRIALS

When you buy new gloves for a specific task, I said you only need to run trials on two or three different kinds of new glove models, along with the incumbent glove. But that assumes you did a rigorous hazard assessment, and *all* the trial gloves meet your new requirements, per task. If you try to run a trial on as many as ten different gloves, you will likely find the logistics a nightmare and the feedback confused. One week is probably a good length of time for a trial. A month is probably too long.

You will need to:

1. Create a glove evaluation form that gathers useful, detailed information, well beyond "I like this glove" or "These gloves suck." Choose your questions carefully, and see the example in Appendix 2A.

2. Select workers to give you balanced feedback, maybe between ten and thirty individuals. A hundred workers will prove too difficult to coordinate. Two or three are generally too few, because you won't get feedback from a wide enough variety of users and situations to be useful.

3. Make sure the trial participants understand the importance of the task. They will be making a decision that will impact the safety of both themselves and their coworkers—a huge responsibility. Timely, honest, usable feedback will be critical. Frame it like, "Here's a choice of three gloves we are considering to replace the existing glove. All of them meet the cut level, puncture level, and impact resistance we think is required for this work. But which do you like best? Which is comfortable and flexible enough? Which has the best grip? We need really detailed, specific feedback on this form so we can get the right glove for everyone working on this equipment."

4. Identify the naysayers, and pull them out for a preparatory conversation. You know who I am talking about—that guy with his arms crossed, who never has a positive thing to say. This person could well kill the whole effort with a bad joke. Pull that guy out, and tell him privately, "Listen, this is really important. I know you've done this for a long time, so I really need your detailed feedback, more than everyone else's. Also please encourage everyone else to take this seriously." Make that guy part of your team.

5. Don't just casually pass out the samples and forms. Hand them out in a formal meeting, and identify someone who will closely monitor the situation, to make sure the gloves get used and the forms filled out. At the meeting remind everyone how vital it is to get the details into the forms: Are the gloves hot? Sweaty? Go over the questions in detail and explain that workers won't be evaluating something like

cut resistance, which reflects a standard, but they will be evaluating dexterity and the general "feeling of protection."

6. Make sure you also ask for unstructured comments, outside of any requirements or standards, like "This glove tends to snag on sharp edges" or, "There's loose material that prevents me from reaching in to fix things." These comments can be vital.

7. Tabulate the data. Then use that data, along with the glove specifications and cost to make a structured, logical decision. You can see a sample tabulation for one glove trial in Appendix 2B.

8. A lot of trouble? You bet. Worth the trouble? Absolutely.

9. *For more information on glove selection, see Appendix 1G for links to online glove selection tools.*

THE GLOVE VALUE DISCONNECT

In chapter four I talked about some of the psychological and social "gaps" between management and workers that work against safety. I want to end this chapter by talking about another kind of gap, which I'll call the "glove value disconnect." It applies specifically to gloves, and it harms both management and workers.

Here's how the disconnect happens:

Management puts a ton of effort and good intention into selecting an expensive glove to protect their workers. Then, to their despair, they see the workers toss the gloves aside when the gloves get just a little dirty, or workers lose the gloves, or take multiple pairs home never to return, or *they just don't wear the friggin' things,* even when badgered. Tens of thousands of dollars may be seen as wasted.

This is especially a problem with seasonal workers or temporary immigrants, who have no apparent long-term investment in the job. Management may go to such workers and say, "Hey, these gloves cost eight dollars a pair! We can't have you going through four pairs a day! If you took care of those gloves, one pair would last a week!" But these words may cause only enmity, or fall on deaf ears. The disconnect gets even worse with a language barrier.

Soon, management may look down from the executive suite and say, "Screw these guys. We try to protect them, but they won't cooperate." Soon, management may switch back to cheap gloves that offer no real protection.

As for the workers, they do not understand that management actually cares, and has provided an expensive glove that needs to be preserved. They also don't perceive management's costs as real, or important—and they see gloves as mere disposable consumables instead of valuable items. Management feels unappreciated, and begins to think of workers as stupid and stubborn.

What's the underlying problem here? *Zero team spirit.*

The workers were probably not involved in glove selection. They never saw the trade-offs and decision-making required to buy those expensive gloves. Management never discussed the overall safety problem with the workers, and workers never felt comfortable sharing their safety concerns with management.

The two parties are operating in separate worlds, without a shared value agreement on the work or on safety.

Gloves are personal. Gloves are expensive. Gloves matter. That means that the selection and deployment of gloves must *always* be part of the overall team effort I described back in chapter four. People value what they help select and what they help control. Bring everyone onto the same team, and the value disconnect will disappear.

What can you do to choose the proper gloves and overcome a value disconnect to protect both your workers and your bottom line?

CHAPTER SEVEN

IN SEARCH OF THE GENUINE HAZARD ASSESSMENT

Plenty of times in earlier chapters I said, "Do this after you do a hazard assessment." The right infrastructure changes, the right signage, the right gloves, the right training: everything depends on a good hazard assessment. But a good hand hazard assessment is not a simple task. It requires not just specific expertise, but a keen awareness of all the cognitive biases and social influences we discussed earlier.

Where to start? How about with a guarantee.

I absolutely guarantee that your workers currently face systematic hand dangers they don't see and you don't see.

After all, that's how the universe plays its little games.

In fact, studies have shown that, in general, workers are only aware of about 45 percent of the hazards they face.[100] Your job is to see *more* risks than they do. Your job is to identify as many of the hidden dangers as possible, *before* they happen. Not *after* they happen. Then make workers aware of each risk, take steps to eliminate or reduce each risk, based on the hierarchy of controls in chapter five.

Does all that seem obvious?

Obviously not, considering how often workers and managers alike say stuff like, "Yeah, I guess that machine could catch a finger, but it's never happened yet."

Or how often, after a hand gets crushed, someone says, "Looking back, I guess it's obvious something like that was just waiting to happen."

DON'T GO IT ALONE

Pretty often a hazard assessment consists of just the safety manager walking through the shop floor with a clipboard, making some notes and writing up a report.

But it is inevitable that a single person, no matter how expert, will miss things.

Also, vitally, workers must feel involved in hazard assessments, to validate them in their eyes, and to get their commitment to changes in behavior to reduce the risk. Note again the "glove value gap" we discussed in the last chapter.

Three or four sets of eyes will see far more, especially if that group includes a mix of experienced workers, experienced managers, and an expert from entirely outside the organization.

A worker will see something you, the safety manager, or the supervisor, will not see. You will see something they don't see.

But the outside expert can also be critical. First, hazard consultants do this all the time, and second, they will be *less subject to the cognitive biases of the people who do the work day in and day out.* A number of companies specialize in full-blown hazard assessments, which go well beyond a narrow "glove assessment" or "signage assessment." These consultants or companies will also suggest infrastructure changes to address the risk—including strategies you may never have considered. A few are listed in Appendix 3.

That means you need to go through the plant with a select team that includes a couple of experienced workers, a supervisor, and an outside expert. You use a checklist and you identify hazards like pinch points in conveyor belts, carrying requirements for sharp objects, lathes, etc.

And you do it more than once.

WHEN AND HOW OFTEN?

A hazard assessment should never be a mere annual event. Stuff changes too often.

Indeed, in some ever-shifting environments, like mines or construction sites—and even in many manufacturing situations—some kind of hand hazard check must occur every single morning. This morning checklist should be conducted by the safety manager in conjunction with supervisors, and the checklist must be updated constantly, as the environment evolves.

New construction site? Machinery relocated? New task? Each change should trigger at least a partial reassessment.

A more comprehensive assessment may occur monthly or quarterly. A responsible company will put in place a strict schedule of these major assessments, coupled with daily or weekly minor assessments.

TIME AND PLACE HAZARDS

When and where matter a lot in hazard assessments.

To correctly see all the hazards, you need to see the operations *actually taking place*, but you also need to see operations during *different shifts*, with *several different workers*, to understand what's actually likely to happen. For example, studies have shown that:

- Accidents are more likely when workers perform a task which is not in their usual list of assignments.
- Accidents are more likely when a machine or tool is performing differently than expected.
- Accidents are more likely about three to four hours into a shift—on a morning shift, for example, there's literally a peak of hand injuries between 10 a.m. and 11 a.m.[101]

Is there a shift with mostly guys under twenty-five? Maybe you should come back and observe then, since they are a higher risk group.

Is there a shift in which newer workers seem unaware of the dangers that have been observed by workers in *another* shift?

Is there a shift in which you've heard that protocol is not being followed, even though other shifts seem to be following it? Specific worker behavior is also part of your hazard assessment.

These kinds of proactive, dynamic observations will be crucial to a genuine assessment.

FINDING POTENTIAL ENERGY

When you and your team head out with those clipboards, you will need to engage both your lizard and your analytic brain, in the ways we first discussed back in chapter four.

As safety expert, Matt Hallowell, puts it, "There are some types of hazards that people will see almost automatically. I mean everybody sees them…then there's a whole category of hazards that are processed by a different part of the brain. These often go unnoticed unless the brain is prompted to look for them. Current [hazard assessment] methods don't prompt people to look there."[102]

Hallowell thinks about hazards as "energy," either potential energy or releasing energy. If you are standing up on a height, you readily see the potential energy of the fall. If you are standing next to a spinning blade, you readily see the releasing energy of the spin. Either way, the danger is immediately obvious to your lizard brain. But potential energy can be hidden, as in a corrosive chemical that looks just like water, or a sharp edge hiding in a pile of debris. And what *exactly* is in those buckets that have been sitting at the edge of the shop floor for the last few months?[103] Hidden dangers require the analytic brain to step back and *consider* before taking action.

As a person doing a hazard assessment, everyone is depending on your analytic brain and the brains you bring with you to see dangers they do not see. They're also depending on you to do your homework on the baseline dangers within your industry (see the section on "Ignoring the Baseline" in chapter three).

Are workers aware of the dangerous nature of all the chemicals they are handling? Are the guys laying the fiberglass insulation aware of the danger of handling the stuff without gloves or inhaling the dust when it's cut? Are the people clearing waste aware of those potential sharps?

All these lie in Hallowell's category of unrecognized potential energy which may only be seen during a focused hazard assessment, or recognized by someone aware of the baseline dangers.

Always remember that workers must do more than follow a protocol like "always wear gloves." They must understand and see the danger themselves. If they do not, that is in and of itself a hazard.

FALSE SECURITY

A major threat to hands comes from equipment which offers the illusion of safety protections, but actually provides little security in practice. A perfect example is the mandatory safety guard on a band saw. At first glance, the guard *apparently* protects the hand from the spinning blade, but it is designed to rise up over a piece of wood as it is fed through the saw. Since workers have their hands on the wood as they maneuver it through the blade, the safety guard will simply rise up over their fingers, too, and protect them not at all.

Indeed, since it often entirely *hides* the spinning saw band, the guard may give the worker a false sense of security, and actually prevent a vital trigger for the lizard brain.

No glove, even chainmail, will fully solve this problem. Is there a tool to push the wood that can keep the worker's hands away from the blade altogether? What combination of new infrastructure and training is needed?

CREATING AND MAINTAINING YOUR CUSTOM CHECKLIST

I've included sample hazard assessment checklists linked in Appendix 3, but you should consider these only a starting point. No general-use checklist will work for every situation, and there's a great danger in going through some generic checklist created by an industry association, or a safety manager at your company ten years ago—or a book like this—and thinking you are done.

You need to construct your own checklist, and you need to update it constantly.

In Appendix 3, you will find an overall Hand Hazard Tracker with multiple tabs, along with a checklist of questions to prompt your assessment of each department. Below you will find a series of steps that walk you through the assessment process. All this will need to be modified for your needs.

STEP 1: DETERMINE YOUR TIMEFRAME

Will a major assessment be run every six months with weekly updates? What makes sense for your company or department?

Major Assessment Schedule: _____

Minor Assessment Schedule: _____

Daily Safety Checks: _____

STEP 2: CHOOSE YOUR ASSESSMENT TEAM

You may have a formal HSE committee to work with, but as we discussed, you need that small but broad team to focus on creating assessments:

Safety Manager: _____

Supervisor: _____

Worker Representatives: _____

_____

Outside Safety Consultant: _____

STEP 3: CREATE YOUR HIGH-LEVEL HAZARD LIST

You can start with the samples in Appendix 3, but you will need to modify it significantly with:

1. What are the baseline hand dangers in your industry? If you're in construction, for example, how are people most

commonly injured by nail guns, and what steps are now being taken to prevent those injuries?

2. What special risks arise within your company? If you're in manufacturing, what are the risks at different stages from raw material to finished product?

3. For the minor assessments: What changed since yesterday? Didn't the guys just rig a winch to haul rocks out of the excavation? Is that winch going to grab a hand?

To create a systematic review, it helps to think about each job as a *process*, through all the stages of the task. But it's also good to run through a list of the types of hand injuries we discussed back in chapter one, and the cognitive biases we identified in chapter three. You can then construct a high-level matrix of processes against hand dangers, like this:

Department	Cuts	Vibration	Chemical	Electric	Heat	Cold	Impact	Puncture	Other
1. Receiving									
2. Assembly									
3. Paint									
4. Inspection									
5. Shipping									

You should then go into more detail within each department down to the steps in each job, like this:

Job Steps-Assembly	Cuts	Vibration	Chemical	ARC	Heat	Cold	Puncture	Other
1. Lift part								
2. Position part								
3. Screw in								
4. Test variance								
5. Polish								

None of these lists can be completed just sitting at a desk in your office. As discussed above, you need to get down into the jobsite multiple times, at different hours, taking into consideration all the factors of time, place, and the mix of people in particular shifts.

STEP 4: CHARACTERIZE RISK

Now that you have overcome your own cognitive biases, considered potential energy as well as releasing energy, talked to the workers, and painstakingly created an inventory of hazards, it is important to get some *priorities* in place. Naturally, I'm not saying that you wouldn't want to fix all the hazards—you absolutely do—but creating a priorities matrix will let you decide which to work on first.

Risk is characterized by the potential severity multiplied by the likelihood the accident could happen. The math is helpful, but if something could kill a worker, you obviously need to think about that first—regardless of the likelihood.

In some jobs, a severity of *five* in the consequences might represent a possible fatality. In others, it might mean loss of a hand.

See Appendix 3 for links to downloadable versions of hazard assessment spreadsheets.

Hazard	Possible consequences	Severity of consequences 1-5 (5 is highest)	Likelihood 1-5 (5 is highest)	Risk Score (0-25) Multiply Severity x Likelihood	Priority to address (high, medium, low)
Moving logs	Serious hand crush injury	4	2	8	Medium
Vibrating equipment	Hand-Arm Vibration Syndrome (HAVS)	3	5	15	High
Table Saws	Severe cuts, loss of fingers	5	3	15	High

STEP 5: EXPLORE HAZARD OPTIONS

Now that you've prioritized risks, it's time to work out ways to eliminate or reduce them, sticking strictly to the hierarchy of controls from chapter five. Take your top priorities and have serious discussions of all possible options with the people who understand the work and the risk best. As you go through the hierarchy, remember always to start at the top, and don't forget that multiple levels and approaches may be needed.

Priority	Hazard	Possible Consequences	Potential Solution Strategies					
			Eliminate	Substitute	Isolate	Engineer	Admin	PPE
1	Vibrating equipment	HAVS					Protocol: must wear anti-vibration gloves	Anti-vibration gloves
1	Table saws	Severe cuts, loss of fingers			Tool to move wood	New guards	Training	
2	Hand crush from moving logs into position	Serious crush injury	Electronic eye and robot arm to eliminate manual positioning				New protocol for warnings	

STEP 6: CREATE AND EXECUTE AN ACTION PLAN

Once you've chosen the best strategies, decide on the next steps and the timeline to implement each step. Remember that every single day a hazard is not addressed is a day someone on your team faces unnecessary risk. Here's an example of a prioritized action plan:

Priority	Hazard	Possible Consequences	Options to Eliminate/ Minimize	Action Decisions	Completed By:
1	Vibrating equipment	HAVS	Mandatory anti-vibration gloves worn for this work. Rotate jobs Change equipment	Mandatory anti-vibration gloves worn for this work. Rotate jobs	May 1
1	Table saws	Severe cuts, loss of fingers	Custom tool to move wood, instead of direct hand application New safety guards Specific safety training with demo	Custom tool to move wood, instead of direct hand application Specific training with demo	May 1
2	Hand crush from moving logs into position	Serious crush injury	New protocol to call "hands clear" before final lowering of log Purchase electronic eye to position logs.	Purchase electronic eye and robot arm to position logs to eliminate manual positioning	August 1

In Appendix 3, and in the download links, you will find more comprehensive spreadsheets that you can modify for your particular situation.

STEP 7: CREATE FOLLOW-UP, MAINTENANCE, AND STATISTICS CHECKLISTS

As you complete each action item, you need to create the follow-up checklists for use by anyone monitoring the hazards you discovered.

Are the robotic arms operating correctly? Are the anti-vibration gloves actually being used? Are they being replaced as needed? These checklists will be a key source of your *leading indicators*, a subject we will explore in depth in chapter nine on metrics. Below you will find a sample maintenance checklist and a suggested method for gathering leading hand-safety indicators for your work, but devising these checklists for your own application will take some serious thought and ingenuity.

Hazard Solution Follow-Up and Maintenance Checklist: Millwork

Hazard	Danger	Solutions	In Place	Maintenance Checks	Check-up Oct 1
Vibrating equipment	HAVS	Mandatory anti-vibration gloves worn for this work. Rotate jobs	May 16	Gloves laundered, replaced regularly Job rotation occurring properly	Need new glove supplier Shortcuts in job rotation, need to address
Table saws	Severe cuts, loss of fingers	Custom tool to move wood, instead of direct hand application Specific training with demo	May 25	Wood-moving tool evaluations, maintenance Observe training	Tool working well, according to mill team. Training sometimes skipped on new employees, need to address
Hand crush from moving logs into position	Serious crush injury	Purchase electronic eye and robot arm to position logs to eliminate manual positioning	August 18	Evaluate robot arm and electronic eye for effectiveness	Danger when equipment jams. Training needed to address

Monthly Hand Safety Leading Indicators

Scored 0-3 (0=Not Happening, 1=Spotty Compliance, 2=Generally Consistent, 3=High Compliance)

Indicator	Oct 1	Nov 1	Jan 1	Feb 1	Score Since Oct 1 (out of 12 possible)
Vibration gloves laundered, replaced regularly	3	2	1	2	8
Vibration tools: job rotation	3	3	3	1	10
Wood-moving tool effectiveness and use	3	3	3	3	12
Table saw training: new employees	3	2	2	1	8
Log positioning robot arm safety	3	2	3	2	10

THE CHALLENGE OF INSTITUTIONAL MEMORY

One of the biggest safety challenges in any industrial setting is *continuity*.

You may go through an elaborate process to identify a specific cut hazard, put in custom safety guards and carefully choose the right gloves—only to have a new supervisor come in, randomly order new gloves when the old ones wear out, and go back to the OEM safety guards when equipment is reordered.

You may not even be around to complain.

Institutional memory depends not on specific people, but on culture and process.

If you succeed in establishing a formal hazard assessment process, along with follow-ups, regularized checklists, and meaningful statistics, you really can succeed in passing down a legacy of safety. Years and years from now, people will be following your process and your standards each time they look at hazards, choose gloves, or install new equipment.

If you depend only on your own expertise, the force of your personality, and your specific relationships with supervisors and management, you may succeed for a time in improving safety, but you will not have changed the culture of your organization, and you will have no impact on workers in future years.

No Shortcuts Based on Your Authority

You may also destroy formal process and continuity if you use your authority to shortcut a hazard assessment and remediation process *which you may yourself have instituted.*

If you say, "Forget all that! Somebody got cut handling glass yesterday! Switch to these new gloves right away!" you may not even be solving the immediate crisis. As we saw in the last chapter, if workers are not involved in assessing the danger and choosing a remedy, such as new gloves, you may be burdening them with gloves they don't value or use, and which might actually make them clumsier when they handle that glass. Even worse, if you teach them to ignore process and passively wait in the future for you or some new executive to rush in with a solution, the team may ignore a worse danger than that sharp glass.

In the interviews for this book, I encountered safety managers who saw carefully built hand-safety programs bulldozed by well-meaning, but over-eager company officers offering instant solutions.

Never forget that when you ignore or destroy process, you damage long-term safety, and you cripple institutional memory. You need a company-specific process to do an injury retrospective, figure out what happened, and come up with ways to fix it. Then you need to stick to that process. This isn't "bureaucracy" it's "long-term thinking."

CHAPTER EIGHT

RETHINKING TRAINING

"The biggest problem with communication is the illusion that it's taken place."

—GEORGE BERNARD SHAW

Safety training often fails.

If you're in the safety business, you probably know that already. You also know that frustrations are part of the game:

"I was on a roll," says a safety trainer. "I was halfway into my speech on gloves and boots and I was being really eloquent, and everyone in the place was nodding and smiling. I was thinking, 'Hey, this is great, I'm really getting through to these guys.' Then, when I pause to take a sip of coffee, a supervisor comes up and says in an undertone, 'Maybe I should just tell you, most of these people don't speak English. They've just learned to nod their heads when a white guy is speaking. Try to hurry it up, because they want to get back to work.'"

"The hardest thing," says another trainer, "is getting someone to believe that it can actually happen to them. Statistics don't seem to have any impact, so I've pretty much stopped citing statistics. Unless they've personally lost a finger, or seen someone lose a finger, they just don't believe it's real. I try to tell them stories like, 'I've seen this. I've actually seen this happen.' I show them horrible pictures. But it's best if someone else in the session decides to stand up, someone they know, someone who's doing the same job as them, and says, 'Yes, here's what I saw. I saw my buddy burn his hands because he wasn't wearing gloves. He was in the hospital for three days.'" This trainer concludes soberly, and a bit resignedly, "I see that counts with them."

"People like me come from a privileged class," says a third, who travels for a professional safety training company. "We're educated. We live in a different world. I show up, I boot up my PowerPoint show, and I say, 'wear your safety equipment.' But I don't know who I am talking to. I have no idea if that guy in the audience is working three construction jobs, has to provide his own equipment, and would never, ever spend the extra money for the right gloves and sleeves and stuff. I don't know whether, if he complained about conditions, he would lose his job that same afternoon, and wouldn't be able to feed his kids the next day. Will he listen to me?"

LOOKING MORE CLOSELY

I sympathize with the plight of these trainers, but I need to say something a bit brutal to them:

These frustrations are all your own fault.

You didn't find out who you were training. You didn't talk to the workers in advance of your session to find out their concerns, identify their known dangers, and learn their experiences.

That means you just plain aren't doing your job.

To the first trainer: I'm sorry, but how can you possibly stare out at an audience of mostly Hispanic workers and not find out if they speak English before you begin?

To the second: Why don't you go canvass workers before you give these talks, to see if they've witnessed horrible accidents on their own equipment? Maybe prep one of them to speak, if they'd be comfortable doing that—and not hope someone stands up spontaneously? And heck, it's possible you're forcing everyone in a room to relive traumatic recent memories of mangled coworkers, every time you show your graphic pictures.

To the third: How could you not take the trouble to learn if the people you are speaking to have to supply their own equipment? Or if they have an established mechanism to report dangers?

The relationship of trainer to trained in an industrial setting is not the relationship of adult to child. Often the trained know more than the trainer, and even when they don't, you absolutely have to find out where they are and what they are thinking before you try to fix their thinking. Workers are never blank slates for your information.

DISCONNECT AT ACME TEXTILES

Let's consider the frustrations of Pete, a hypothetical trainer for Acme Textiles, which has seen an alarming number of injuries on their WeaveBot equipment.

At 9 a.m., Pete holds a formal session in which he spends forty minutes explaining how to handle the WeaveBot Triple Yarn Spindle safely, and especially how to drop the clutch in the way recommended by the manufacturer, so as not to pinch fingers. Finally he emphasizes that everyone in the shop should wear their new No. 4 abrasion-resistant gloves when performing this task, due to the recent spate of serious abrasion injuries.

Then lo and behold, come 2 p.m., Pete tours the floor and sees everyone handling the WeaveBot the same dangerous way they've always handled it. They're not even wearing the damn gloves!

Pete thinks, "What, are these people stupid? Reckless? Were they just not listening? Not watching my slides?"

Next time, if Pete's lucky, someone will come up to him after his lecture and say, "Um, excuse me, I didn't want to interrupt during the session, but I can't really handle the spindle with that new kind of glove. It's too thick to adjust the controls, and I'm worried it will get caught in the flywheel. Also, the clutches on half those machines are broken, so we usually have to just stop the flywheel with our hands."

Of course, next time, no one will be listening to Pete anyway, since he's so clearly ignorant.

TRAINING IS *COOPERATION*, NOT *COMMUNICATION*

I'd like to say that Pete would be an extreme example, but his training mistakes are all too common:

1. He observed the behavior of employees, but he didn't ask them *why* they were handling the spindle as they did, what they currently considered normal and safe, and what they saw as the real dangers.
2. He didn't check on the actual *condition* of the machinery, and how that led to unsafe work strategies.
3. He didn't talk to the workers to get their feedback on the best approach *in their circumstances* (Glove or no glove? Manufacturer-recommended process or not?).
4. He didn't see that his job was not to lecture *to* the employees, but to work *with* the employees.
5. He failed to establish credibility and trust with the workers before the lecture. Indeed, he sacrificed critical credibility and trust which will be extremely difficult for him to regain.

Like the other trainers I mentioned, Pete approached the workers as one would approach a child: as if he just naturally knew better because he was educated, had read the manuals, and had carefully researched the No. 4 abrasion glove. Those are all good things, but he never realized that *effective training is a form of cooperation, not a form of communication.*

Pete probably obtained the buy-in of executive management on his original PowerPoint and training approach. And why wouldn't they sign off? His presentation looked pretty, it addressed the issue, and it followed a clear communications format. No doubt no one from the executive suite ever went to monitor the results.

If Pete had never toured the floor at 2 p.m., he would have gone home and slept well, thinking he'd delivered something valuable to those workers.

SAFETY IS RELATIVE

The first psychological problem faced by anyone trying to train for safety is pretty basic:

Safety is a relative term.

What Jill considers hand-safe behavior, Jack may not. What Jack considers totally mandatory, Jill may consider highly optional.

Our personal ideas of safety are formed not by any scientific risk analysis, but by our background, culture, job experience, skill level, accidents witnessed, and on and on. Importantly, as we also discussed in chapter four, what's considered *safe* is often simply what's considered *normal*. Regardless of whether an outside observer would consider our actions safe at all.

If workers at Acme Textile see it as *normal* to stop the flywheel with their hand, then that behavior will, over time, come to equal *safe* in their minds—even if an outside observer can see that the behavior is highly dangerous. Indeed, since the spindle clutches were unreliable, they may have felt it unsafe to use the clutch at all, or bother reading the manufacturer's other instructions.

If Pete had sat down with some experienced workers before introducing the new gloves and the related training, they could have discussed how to create a *new, safer normal*—which might, by the way, have included fixing all the broken clutches on the spindles.

Later, at the actual safety lecture, these same highly credible workers could *themselves* have demonstrated this new normal to the others, and then modeled that same behavior throughout the day and beyond. Because the training and a change in work norms came from a reliable source, people would listen. Soon, no one would even remember the bad old way of doing it.

No PowerPoint needed.

Bottom line: You must achieve agreement on what is safe, and you must redefine safe as normal. That means it's the job of a trainer not to deliver information, but to shift the very idea of "normal." Such a shift can only be accomplished by close, credible cooperation with workers as adults.

THE TROUBLE WITH ON-THE-JOB MENTORS

Since hand-safety training is a relationship, not an information delivery system, it matters a lot who does the training.

Really, really a lot.

At plenty of jobsites, the training of new employees consists of telling a recruit to follow an experienced worker around for a few days in a mentoring relationship. If your mentor is Harry, you'll learn whatever Harry knows about the job and whatever Harry knows about safety. Then maybe you'll get a safety brochure to take home or a video to watch. Then maybe you'll hear a toolbox talk by your supervisor once a month, which hopefully includes some hand-safety information.

The brochure will likely never get read, or it will be so generic as to be useless for your particular job. The video will be silly, and even more generic. Depending on the rhetorical skills of the team boss, his toolbox talk may or may not have an impact on you.

But Harry! Those few days with Harry may determine the course of the rest of your life. If Harry wears gloves, you'll wear gloves. If he doesn't wear gloves, you won't wear gloves. If he runs a safety check on equipment before using it, you'll run a safety check. If he switches on the drill without the safety shield, you'll switch on the drill without the safety shield.

Even if Harry proves to be highly hand-safety conscious, Harry only knows what he knows. Harry probably has no idea of industry baselines, the history of injuries in these tasks at the company, available glove options, or all the other things that should shape safety decisions and training.

If you are a newbie recruit, how are you going to learn to be safer than Harry?

GABE HANDLES GLASS BAREHANDED

Here's an on-the-job mentoring story from one of my company's reps:

"We went down to this glass parts factory and asked about their safety training protocol. Basically, new recruits were given a safety brochure, and then assigned to follow a guy we'll call Gabe around for two days, because Gabe was one of their most experienced workers. After two days with Gabe, you were on your own to do the job.

"We went and met with Gabe, who was a friendly enough guy, and no doubt very experienced. But Gabe scared the hell out of us as a 'mentor' in the first thirty seconds of our conversation.

"As part of their job, the employees often had to move panes of glass from a cutting machine, then through a chemical bath. When we met, Gabe held up his hands to show us his many scars, and immediately said, 'Yeah, I've sliced myself up pretty badly a few times. I just hate wearing gloves. They get all sweaty. My hands are pretty tough, though.' We could see that he considered these scars as a kind of badge of honor.

"We watched Gabe move the glass sheets through some kind of burnt orange-colored chemical bath, the exact contents of which Gabe did not know. Sometimes he'd start with gloves, but then take them off because they didn't have enough grip for the job. Then he'd literally move the glass through the bath barehanded, and just wipe his hands off on a towel. He introduced us to one of his young recruits who had, indeed, cut his hands while they were bare in the chemical bath just a few days before—allowing God knows what chemicals into his system. Basically, we were horrified by what Gabe and the entire company considered *normal*."

Is this your training method? Do you know what your experienced mentors are actually passing on to new workers? Bad safety practices are like viral infections; they get passed on easily.

THE TROUBLE WITH SAFETY TALKS

Now let's get to structured hand-safety talks, whether delivered formally in a classroom setting or delivered casually on the job as "toolbox talks"—either by a designated safety trainer or a team supervisor.

Once again, who gives the talk matters as much or more than what's in the talk.

Does the person have credibility? Have they been there and done that? Is the person actually knowledgeable about gloves, baseline industry dangers, baseline industry safety practices, current safety issues at the company? Is the person willing to go down on the floor and discuss hand-safety issues with the workers and do an assessment before finalizing the content of their talks? Will the workers actually talk to this person? Do they speak well? Are they passionate about their responsibility, or were they moved into safety training only because they were failing at something else?

CLARITY ON GOALS

Just as importantly, does the person giving the safety talk have a conflict in goals?

If I'm a team supervisor and I have heavy pressure to meet production demands, including getting new recruits up to speed quickly, what priority am I going to place on hand-safety training? During training, what am I secretly communicating with my tone and gestures? As we discussed in chapter four, a great deal can be communicated in a tone of voice, a glance, or a shrug:

Will a supervisor indicate with a sly grin that gloves are actually optional, even while he or she is saying they are mandatory?

And of course, does this person *actually* practice hand safety themselves on the job? How do you know what hand-safety measures they actually practice? Have you gone to see?

If the presenter is a professional trainer or a company executive, what are their goals? Their goals must not be "check the safety box" or "present a lot of great statistics and impress the audience that they've done the homework."

Their goal must be, "create safety."

CREDIBILITY COUNTS

One of the mistakes we discussed in chapter two was using non-credible trainers.

You don't have to be an actual worker at a plant, you don't have to know anyone there personally, but you do have to be perceived as someone who has seen and cared about hand-safety issues *firsthand*.

Sometimes establishing credibility requires as little as giving one's qualifications, then telling a personal story like the one found in the sidebar later in this chapter. (See also rule #3 under my golden rules, below.)

But there's more. A credible trainer will be perceived as a member of the "fraternity" of industrial workers, not industrial managers. He or she won't waste the time of workers with irrelevant detail. Won't give rules without explanations for the rules. Will be sure that real-world experience backs up every prescription for safety. Will acknowledge that he or she maybe doesn't know as much as the workers about certain details.

Five minutes in, your credibility on these points will have been judged. Maybe two minutes in. The trainer must show that he or she "gets it." And fast.

At the very least, make sure you are introduced by a credible person in the workplace. Don't just show up and introduce yourself. A little of their credibility will rub off on you.

BORING IS A FORM OF FAILURE

Hand-safety training absolutely cannot be boring. I'm sorry, but audience interest is not a "nice to have;" it's a "must-have." If people are not interested and engaged in what you are saying, they are not going to retain the information—it's that simple.

I can't believe how difficult it is to convey this simple truth to safety managers the world over, who usually seem to accept the idea that safety is inevitably a dull topic. Every one of these people should be able to look back on their own school experience to understand how that attitude causes them to fail in their duty to train. In school, you crammed boring information to pass a test, then you forgot it; you retained interesting material, presented by engaging teachers, for life.

Remember?

Again and again, however, working men and women with a vital interest in their own safety, who are out in dangerous roadways, down in mines, in the bellies of airplanes, or sailing at sea—are subjected to tedious PowerPoint slides with hundreds of bullet points, or safety videos with actors in slow motion accompanied by a monotonous voiceover. Over time, workers learn to snooze through these shows and ignore them. Let me put this in bold type:

The dullness of presentations presents an active danger. Boring is a form of failure.

Here are some secrets to stop being boring:

1. *Develop a personal story* you can tell to make a vital personal connection between yourself, your audience, and the material. It can be about a relative, a friend, or a coworker—but you have to have a personal connection and really care about the story. It doesn't have to be 100 percent relevant to the situation, but your personal involvement with safety will create automatic interest and a common bond with listeners. I give a couple examples in the sidebar below.

2. *Remember that words on screens suck.* More words on screens suck even more. The human mind is simply incapable of retaining lots of bullet points, not to mention the problem of workers with poor language skills. It's okay to do some (not all) PowerPoint, but the show should be 99 percent pictures, with maybe one or two words per slide: "Pinching Danger" or "Right Way" and "Wrong Way." Remember also that if you don't have words on the screen, workers will have to listen to you talk. *The stuff on the screen should just catch interest and illustrate what you are saying, never substitute for what you are saying or discussing or demonstrating.*

3. *Photos work.* Yes, gruesome photos, sometimes, and used with the care we discussed in chapter three. But photos of doing the job right and wrong, are crucial for sure. Videos of donning and doffing gloves correctly when using dangerous chemicals, but without stupid voiceovers. Just the pics and video in the background, as you talk and engage. Photos of "near misses" can be particularly effective, as I discuss in a section below. But make sure always to leave the audience with a positive, "right way" image.

4. *Humor works.* Beyond holding interest, good humor is *disarming*, it reduces objections. Good humor also puts you on the *same side* as your audience—"we are laughing together."

Our trainers have used any number of humorous videos to good effect, even when dealing with very serious topics. Funny stock photos and cartoons work too—we use them all the time in our training materials and on our website. Humor must, of course, always be used with caution: no politics, religion, sexist, or sexual orientation jokes. Humor must also be universal—something everyone can relate to. That means you should use clips from popular TV shows, not something obscure.

5. *Variety is mandatory.* Far too often, trainers reuse the same infographics, the same statistics, and the same photos over and over again to make the same point. Even if the audience has changed, this will eventually dull your own presentation skills. As every performer and teacher knows, you must be willing to take risks with new material, try new approaches, and engage your audiences in different ways or you will become stale over time. Often, this means introducing material which is not strictly relevant to your audience, just to get their attention. For example, expert trainer, Delaney King, who I quote in the sidebar below, sometimes employs rather shocking humor, like an out-there video about teaching safety to high school students in shop class.[104]

6. *Create a conversation.* Ask workers about glove use in a group setting. Get their feedback, their tips and tricks to stay safe. Get them telling their personal safety stories. Get everyone past their discomfort of discussing safety in a group and they will become genuinely engaged, maybe even proud of their contributions to everyone's well-being. If you are doing all the talking, you are doing something wrong.

7. *Remember to keep it short…*

8. *…And don't pack it all into one show.* The human mind can only absorb so much in one sitting. Presenting fifty bullet points in sixty minutes makes it unlikely that people will

remember even five of those points. Giving a solid discussion of five points in ten minutes, with another ten minutes of discussion, makes it pretty likely that people will remember those five points.

9. *Be willing to change.* Most safety trainers get into a rut. Often they're completely unaware that no one's listening to them. If your message isn't getting across, you need to be honest with yourself and your audience. You need to be willing to say, "Hey, you guys don't seem to be getting this, let's try it a different way."

10. *... Which means you must critique yourself.* Videotape yourself giving a presentation and force yourself to watch it. Are you mumbling? Being dismissive of others? Repeating yourself? Going on and on and on? What can you do to shorten it, tighten it, spice it up? I guarantee the first time you do this you will be shocked at how boring you are.

THE CRUCIAL PERSONAL STORY

Safety expert Delaney King often trains trainers, and she well knows that training is more about relationship than information delivery. "I tell people they absolutely have to develop a personal story about safety that they can share with an audience. Actually, they need both a negative and a positive story, a disaster and a problem solved.

"The stories truly have to be personal, not second or third hand: A *relative* was injured. You *spoke* to the victim. It happened in *your* factory. It mattered to *you.* Personal stories create an emotional bond between you and your audience, but they also create 'reality.' You become living proof, right in front of your audience, that such accidents actually happen, and aren't just statistics or stories about 'others.' Here's a story I use again and again when I speak:

"We have a neighbor down the road. He's a minister and he's got seven kids. A little while back, this minister took up carpentry as a hobby. He was going to make all kinds of furniture in his garage. I told him, 'Hey, you should invest in a good pair of gloves. I'll even give you a pair to borrow.' But he was like, 'No, no, I'm fine, I don't need a pair of gloves.' Naturally, I persisted, 'Well, you've got some pretty serious tools there, you know? There are these amazing cut-resistant gloves now, they're really flexible and all.' But he shut me down. 'No, it's fine,' he said.

"A week or so later I get a text from his wife: 'How long do you have to reattach fingers if they get cut off?' I'm looking at this text, and I'm thinking 'Jesus, is this something you text somebody?' My husband is an advanced care paramedic, so I call him and he says, 'Well, not very long. You've got to pick them up and put them in an ice bag and get right to the hospital with them.'

"I talk the minister's wife into all this. She's just had a baby two weeks earlier, by the way, but she packs up the baby and some of the kids and takes the minister to the hospital with his three severed fingers on ice.

"Now, we live in a small, rural town with a small hospital. At the hospital, the doctor says, 'I'm not a plastic surgeon. We don't have one here. I'll reattach what I can. Let's see, hmmm, I'll just take the skin and flip it over the end and sew it off, maybe, and make what I can out of what's left here.' The wife was horrified at his ignorance, but what could she do?

"Later, the minister goes to a real plastic surgeon in a bigger town, and the surgeon says, "Good Lord, was the doctor drunk? This is terrible. The surgeon tries to reconstruct the hand as best he can, but he's missing some key bits and pieces and there's not a lot he can do. As for the minister, it's not just the missing fingers, he's on weeks of opioids. They become addictive. He has psychological issues that result—truly his entire life is changed.

"So what happened that day in the garage? The minister was pushing a piece of wood through a table saw, and he reached over the blade to grab the wood from the other side, but his hand slipped and got caught in the blade, and in an instant, three fingers were gone. Blood spurting. The fingers on the other side of the room. Panicking as he runs to his wife. Why? First, because he wouldn't spend ten or fifteen bucks on good gloves. Or for heaven's sake borrow them from me. Second, because he somehow didn't think that such a thing could happen to him. He could never imagine it happening to *him*.

"*That's when I look out meaningfully into my audience.*

"Then I tell my positive story. Sometime later, my husband was at work making mantles. He's pushing one through a blade, and it slipped, and his hand rode right over a spinning blade—but he'd remembered about our friend the minister, and so my husband was wearing the right protective gloves. And because he was wearing the right gloves, his hand bounced right off the blade. He showed me the glove that night, and I could see where it had been scored by the blade. But his hands were fine. Absolutely fine. We stared at the glove together. 'Without that glove,' he said, 'you can see how the blade would have torn through two of my fingers, right here.'

When Delaney tells that story, she may be talking to a road crew that never uses table saws—but it doesn't matter. She's established a bond, a reality, and a meaningful context for everything else she's about to tell them: *It can happen to anyone. I saw that for myself. I'm here as proof. But it's not hopeless. If you take the right steps, you can protect yourself.*

CANNED SHOWS AND TURNKEY PROGRAMS

You will find a huge number of hand-safety shows, training materials, and "turnkey programs" available out there from third parties. Some include just online modules and some include presenters who come onsite, and even do safety assessments. Many of these presenters will be highly knowledgeable, and many will be talented at public speaking—perhaps more talented than your own people. Certainly any outside consultant should be certified by the American Society of Safety Professionals. You will find some links in Appendix 5.

I suggest you think about these programs the same way you think about buying clothing on the internet:

1. You will learn a lot and get ideas just by looking through these programs, and sampling them, but you may ultimately find that you need to put together your own wardrobe, in person.
2. You may buy a bunch of clothes off a website and find that only a few pieces fit well, and the rest need to be sent back.
3. You may buy a few basic necessities online, but ultimately you will probably need to customize the accessories and add on personal items—as pre-selected ensembles will never completely do the job.
4. Would you buy jeans on the internet and have them shipped

to your daughter across the country, then never check back with her to see if they fit? Far too often, executives will select a third-party "hand-safety training program" and impose it on remote sites without getting any input up front or feedback down the line.

5. Would you buy a *complete wardrobe* for your daughter off the internet, then check the CYA box in your mind that says, "Okay, I've done everything I can for her?" I don't think so.

6. Wouldn't you rather establish a relationship with a really knowledgeable salesperson at a boutique who could measure you and help you pick out just the right thing?

Ultimately, canned programs can be great starting points, and can provide a solid foundation for your own efforts—but it's impossible for any of them to achieve the *relationship* goals of a serious training program or fit exactly to the custom needs of your shop.

Be especially wary of programs that promise to "change your company's safety culture" or perform other magic tricks in a short space of time. A third party can help guide you, but the hard work of changing a company culture must come from the top to bottom commitment we discussed in chapter four.

Too often, my team and I have seen executives who really wanted to see a change in their hand-safety record, but didn't want to get personally involved—like by showing up at safety committee meetings or insisting that the entire organization become engaged in the effort. Instead, these folks contract with third-party safety training companies, turn them loose, and figure they've done their job.

Sorry, not gonna work.

Do I believe that third-party materials, trainers, and programs can add huge value to your hand-safety training efforts? Absolutely—and full disclosure, my company offers such programs. Do I think you should proceed with caution and always remember that you bear ultimate responsibility for the outcome? Absolutely.

I TOOK TOO LONG IN THE JOHN

"A woman came up to me after I spoke at a safety conference in Las Vegas. I'll call her Crissy. She'd been a safety trainer at a big factory for about four months, and I asked her what brought her to this kind of work. 'Honestly,' she says, 'I was the last person to a meeting, so I got picked. Before this, I was the office manager.' 'Seriously?' I said. 'Yup. I took too long in the john and when I got to the meeting, my boss says, "Hi Crissy. Now you're our safety person." I honestly said I had no background or experience in safety, but my boss says I shouldn't worry because he's sending me for a train-the-trainer session in Vegas. Plus he gave me a big stack of binders that the last safety person bought for the company. So here I am. But I really don't want this job.'

"'Great,' I think, 'just imagine the powerful training she's going to deliver to people out there working with dangerous tools and machinery.'"—Delaney King, Safety Expert

TRAINING NEWBIES IS DIFFERENT

Training a new recruit is different than training veterans. The trainer must not only ensure that skills training is solid and safety training is solid, *but also that the culture of the company is passed on in a positive way.*

The first days, the first hours, even the first minutes of any raw recruit's time in a job or on a worksite are crucial. Humans are naturally on high alert as they enter a new environment, and they will be looking for clues to how they should behave. Do the veterans follow rules? Do they cut corners? Is the company line just bull? Newbies will draw rapid, first impression conclusions, which are likely to stick with them for the rest of their time at the company.

As a trainer, you have a crucial responsibility to control who newbies interact with as mentors (remember "Gabe," above), and you must give newbies a clear message on company safety culture—possibly with the addendum that *they must follow policy regardless of what they see others doing.*

For a trainer, passing along a company's safety culture is a crucial, but difficult task. Most, however, don't understand the problem at all.

Try asking a trainer, "What is your company's safety culture?" and you will be shocked at how many cannot even formulate an answer. You need a clear story you can tell eye-to-eye with a new recruit—an official, carefully rehearsed, and logical story which does not suffer from the "reality gap" I described back in chapter four.

When you are presenting to a group that includes both newbies and veterans, you also need to have a few veterans you can call upon to publicly share stories in a way which will *reinforce your culture message:* "Vanessa, can you tell that story about the wrench slippage accident again, and how it was handled? I want these new folks to hear that story." Indeed, company lore on accidents—policies followed and especially accidents averted— may be crucial in acculturating a new generation.

THE ROI OF HAND-SAFETY TRAINING

It's not hard to demonstrate the ROI of hand-safety training—both for safety and for the bottom line.

For example, in 2014 Alta Steel participated in the Superior Glove Advocate Hand Protection Program, with goals to: 1) Reduce hand and arm injuries; 2) Reduce overall glove and safety costs; and 3) Reduce redundancy and ensure that the right glove was being used per task. Our territory manager got them to stop letting individual employees choose their own, usually "general purpose" gloves. Everyone was required to switch to task-specific gloves with serious-cut protection, and the change was backed up with hand-safety training. Both costs and injuries dropped dramatically:

Glove spending fiscal 2014: $333,304

Glove spending fiscal 2015: $175,714

That's a reduction of 47 percent!

Hand injuries fiscal 2014: 57

Hand injuries fiscal 2015: 9

That's a reduction of 84 percent!

GOLDEN RULES OF PRESENTATIONS

Here are some golden rules for group training presentations—beyond not being boring. Violate them at your peril and the peril of your workers. You will find some links to sample hand-safety curriculums and materials in Appendix 5.

1. DO A NEEDS ASSESSMENT BEFORE WASTING EVERYONE'S TIME

Never do training for the sake of training. You need to know precisely what the hazards are in a given situation, and precisely what training needs to be provided—and not one ounce more. When you waste people's time you lose more than time, you lose their respect and you lose their attention when it really matters.

Doing a proper needs assessment means much more than just talking to a supervisor and asking "What do these guys need to learn to be safer?" It means running a genuine hazard assessment as described in chapter seven, and pairing it with a training action plan, broken down into manageable bits of information.

Assume that there are plenty of hazards and training lapses which supervisors have ignored or never even noticed.

TRAINING FOR REAL PROBLEMS

A supervisor at a construction site shares this story:

"One day a worker was walking extremely slowly, and truly slowing everyone down. I went up to him a little annoyed, and said, 'You know, you need to pick up the pace. We've got a lot to do here.' The guy just nodded, but he didn't speed up, and all day I found myself giving him grief—until I noticed he was actually limping. It turns out that early in the day another worker had put a nail through this guy's foot with a nail gun. The poor guy had just pulled the nail out, wrapped his foot, and kept working—afraid that if he went to a hospital, he'd lose a day of wages, it might endanger his job, or even threaten his immigration status.

"I realized then that we had to provide first aid right onsite, and not ask people to go to the doctor all the time, because they just wouldn't go. We started bringing a nurse onsite every day. We did nail gun safety training, but we also realized that we couldn't just let everyone know the nurse was around. We had to do a whole lot more training about how to handle an injury, about not powering through an injury, about how it was really okay to take the afternoon off if you were injured, and about exactly how to get help from the nurse—all to make *these particular guys* comfortable."

Importantly, this supervisor did not go to his upper management and ask, "What kind of training should I provide workers?" He saw what needed to be changed, what training was needed to support it, and he made it happen.

2. GET BUY-IN AND LINKAGE

Good training is never an isolated event. You need to coordinate your presentations with overall safety initiatives through the company, with accurate hazard assessments, with simultaneous infrastructure changes, and more.

Training supports overall hand-safety efforts, it does not replace those efforts.

That means getting management buy-in and cooperation at

every necessary level, above and below your own. Otherwise, whatever brilliant work you do in your presentation will be out of context to the overall work and safety efforts of the company, and will ultimately be lost in the background noise of the shop.

3. THE TRAINING ENVIRONMENT MATTERS, A LOT

It matters where you do your training.

If you decide to give everyone a treat by pulling them off the floor and bringing them up to a boardroom, serving them a sushi lunch, handing them notepads, and impressing them with how seriously management takes safety, you're crippling your effort before it's begun.

Why? Everyone will just be uncomfortable, maybe even annoyed in the executive suite. The disjunction between the clean order of the boardroom and the messy shop floor will be distracting and counterproductive. You're taking people from the place where they feel comfortable speaking to a place where they figure no one wants them to speak.

And don't think for a minute anyone's going to be taking notes.

It's much better to go down to the shop floor and say, "Hey, let's pull up some five-gallon pails to sit on, and let's talk about hand safety. I brought some sandwiches."

This brings the power back to the audience, because that's where they thrive, where they are comfortable, and where they are assumed to be the experts.

You might also use a break room which is familiar to everyone, somewhere people can easily come and go if they need to, use the restroom without causing a disturbance, and so forth. Yes, provide snacks—but something familiar to your audience. Snacks break the ice, and everyone likes to do something with their hands while listening.

Take it to them, on their ground. Use their language, let them tell their stories. Oh, and listen to their jokes, no matter how bad or how blue they may be.

4. JUSTIFY YOUR EXISTENCE

You need to do two things when you start a training session. And you need to do them in the first two minutes, tops. If people don't know you, you first need to establish your credibility—yes, that means *briefly* mentioning your certificates in safety, your background in the work, etc. Second, you need to justify the subject you are about to present, and the way you are about to do it.

Why? Because workers are used to management wasting their time with useless training by people who have no understanding of the real issues.

In your *very, very brief* introductory remarks, you need to explain exactly why this training is being presented, and how it was researched: "We've been seeing an uptick in abrasion injuries. We looked into some of the reasons, researched some studies, looked at what people were doing on the shop floor, and we talked to a glove company. Here's what we learned."

Another piece of good advice from a trainer is to ask the audience, "What one thing do you think we should discuss today, that might not come up? What hand-safety issue is worrying you?" This trainer says he'll even put up a whiteboard, and write down a checklist of things people call out. That way they understand that the session is interactive and cooperative—so it's not all on him to make the session work, they need to make it work too.

HERE'S WHY I'M TAKING YOUR TIME

Here's a tale from an experienced glove trainer about justifying her existence.

"One time when I was training at a plant, one of the guys was standing there with his arms crossed, looking skeptical. He wouldn't engage, wouldn't answer any direct questions, even.

"I asked him, 'Is there something wrong?' And he comes back, 'This is just a total waste of my time. I don't know why we have to take these stupid training sessions. Okay, so we should wear gloves. We know we should wear gloves.'"

"'Have you ever had a hand injury here?' I asked. 'Yeah, one time I burnt my hands handling the liquid nitrogen. You know, a cold burn.' In fact, it had been a pretty bad burn. He was wearing gloves, but the liquid nitrogen was so cold it had fused the gloves to his hands and to the container he was holding. He'd been rushed to the hospital.

"'Do you think training could have helped?'

'No, it was the gloves' fault. They were lousy gloves.'

'He used the wrong gloves. He just grabbed some old gloves instead of the cold protection gloves, that's what happened,' piped up his supervisor.

"So I said, 'We're using your time today so that you know the difference between the kinds of gloves, and what's right for what. So that you and others don't accidentally pick up the wrong kind of glove again. I'm hoping that's worth a half hour of your time.'

"But it was *my* fault, the way the whole thing went down. If I had taken the trouble to talk to the workers before, gotten their stories, learned their issues, I could have justified my existence far more quickly and effectively than with that confrontation. And of course, I never should have engaged with this person in front of the group.

"Since that event, I now automatically look for the skeptical people in the audience, the ones standing there with their arms crossed, clearly annoyed. During a break, I'll take them aside and ask for their advice: 'What do you think it's most important for me to cover, here? Do you think I'm focusing on the right stuff?' People love to give advice, and if I get them engaged, they'll bring others along, too. If at all possible, I'll call on that person for a response in the second half of my talk."

5. NEVER TALK ABOUT "STUPID"

When you are training, you can think you are being adult and casual by saying things like, "Let's be smart, not stupid out there." Or "This is just common sense, don't be an idiot." When you do that, however, you immediately throw up a wall between yourself and your audience. Never, ever talk about smart vs. stupid.

Part of implying your audience is stupid, by the way, is to present canned safety material, which has not been customized for the specific work and circumstances of the shop. Immediately, your audience will feel that they are being treated like grammar school kids.

And, of course, never correct people's English or their grammar in a training session. It's disrespectful. Always remember, your English may be better, but that guy knows how to drive a forklift backwards without killing anybody. Could you do that?

6. DEAL DIRECTLY WITH LANGUAGE AND CULTURAL ISSUES

Yes, I know I've brought this up before. But if half of your workers speak Spanish much better than they speak English, you better have an interpreter standing next to you.

Understanding cultures matters, too. If you're presenting in Japan, be aware that you may have a hard time getting anyone in the audience to speak up and contradict something the boss said. Ever.

Generations and Genders Matter, Too

Part of knowing your audience is knowing their generational and gender makeup. These things change fast, but as of this writing...

Baby Boomers tend to like a traditional classroom setting, blackboard and all. They will often sit and listen to a teacher respectfully.

Millennials tend to resent being seated in a classroom manner.

They want to move around, form groups, and ask a lot of questions, including questioning your authority.

Women are less likely to speak up and give a public opinion.

Bottom line? Be aware that in any mix of people you may need to deal with their different ways of behaving in a group. Try to bring everybody into the conversation, and don't get flustered.

Don't be dismissive of these concerns. Getting through to people is your *job.*

7. USE HORRIBLE PICTURES CAUTIOUSLY OR NOT AT ALL

As you design your curriculum, you will want to reread chapter three about the psychology of safety. When you do, pay special attention to the section on fear. In that section, I talk a lot about the proper and improper uses of fear, and how you must always proceed with caution when showing things like bloody pictures of mangled hands or videos of fake hands being torn up in a shredder. You must understand your audience, and if they *want* to see stuff like that. You may be triggering PTSD in people who just witnessed something similar.

Must Be Completely Relevant

In any case, a graphic image must relate directly to the work at hand. Not surprisingly research shows it's far more effective if you can say, "This picture shows an injury that happened on this machine that you will be using."[105]

You will have to gauge your audience, try different tactics, and be ready to pivot when one approach does not work.

8. DISCUSS NEAR MISSES

Trainers have found that "near miss" stories can be more effective than tragic stories in triggering alertness for both the lizard and analytic brains.

If you show a picture of a grinning guy holding a glove that was partway cut through by a spinning blade, you can often get through to an audience and cause real changes in behavior—like wearing gloves.

Why? Because the picture or the story proves the reality of the danger while preventing the recoil and denial that tragedy can cause: *This almost happened. It could happen to you. Be like this happy person, wear your gloves, and you can smile afterwards.*

Now you're creating positive motivation, instead of negative recoil.

Then ask for people to tell their own stories of wearing and not wearing gloves, and the injuries they narrowly avoided. People love to tell near miss stories.

9. INFOGRAPHICS WORK

I said before that words on screens suck. Well, so do numbers. Infographics, in which numbers are changed into cartoons, seem to work far better in proving the reality of statistics to a skeptical or inattentive audience.

A good infographic takes something complex and makes it simple and immediate. Score one for the trainer.

Infographics can then back up the near miss stories you just told, with statistics: *One in four people who don't wear gloves doing your specific work get seriously injured on the job.* Show the one person lined up with three others in a cartoon.

10. STORIES WORK EVEN BETTER

I talked about using your personal stories and gathering stories from your audience, but it's important to remember in your golden rules that stories are not a "nice to have" they're a "must have." Stories help people relate to reality, and they're an important way that people make decisions: "This happened to Carla, so I'd better change my ways."

Indeed, according to the trainers we interviewed, *stories* about incidents are often more effective than *photos* of incidents. Why? Because, as we discussed under rule #6 above, thanks to the media it's becoming harder to escape the reality of a story than it is to ignore a fearful image.

Begin thinking of stories as more than illustrations, and start thinking of them as "social learning." Stories have always been the way the human herd has passed on knowledge. Not PowerPoint.

11. GET PHYSICAL

Imagine trying to teach someone to ride a bicycle using words and pictures, instead of demonstrating how to ride, and getting them to try it themselves.

Real-world demonstrations are a hundred times better than pictures and a thousand times better than words. You create something much better than knowledge, you create a visual memory—and if they get to do it themselves, you create a muscle memory, too.

Pick up a cheap pair of gloves and cut through them with a knife. Show how hard it is to cut through a cut-resistant glove—not impossible, but much more difficult.

Stand next to a rotating piece of machinery and show how easily it can grab a piece of clothing—like a glove or scarf you hold out too close. Let people see the grab happen, and imagine the consequences.

12. VERIFY THAT PEOPLE ACTUALLY GOT TRAINED

How do you know if your words are getting through?

Remember that training is different than education. Education is about transferring a body of knowledge. Training is about changing people's behavior. If there's no change, there has been no training, regardless of how many slides were presented.

During a session, you can tell if you have accomplished education. Only later can you verify that training occurred.

On the Spot Verification

For starters, you absolutely need a way to find out if you are getting through to your audience, right on the spot. It's not enough to pause every now and then and ask, "Is everybody getting this?" then wait for everyone to nod their heads.

You're not going to give some childish quiz to your audience—a quiz which would in itself be pretty meaningless. Nevertheless, you need to devise ways of verifying a transfer of learning. That means asking questions like:

- *Tell me how you're going to apply this when you get back to your job tomorrow?*
- *Tell me how this will make you safer?*
- *Can you demonstrate this new technique for me right now?*
- *Can you summarize back what I just said?*
- *Can you teach this to Jim over there?*
- *Is there something I'm missing in this demonstration?*

In other words, not yes or no questions, but probing questions and demonstrations of knowledge. These questions will also help at least a little to see if you have changed *attitudes* about hand safety. You can tell by the enthusiasm of answers—or the skepticism.

If no one can answer probing questions, or demo back what you've been showing, you know you're not getting anywhere. Challenge your audience and challenge yourself. It's okay to say things like, "If you can't tell me how this will change what you are doing, I'm obviously not doing my job here."

Follow-Up Metrics

As part of developing your curriculum, you also need to define the metrics you will use to measure training success—a week later, a month later, a year later.

Did the training stick? How exactly will you know? A month later, are all the new techniques passed on to new hires? Are workers having any issues with techniques that were demonstrated? Have they devised new techniques? Are the same kinds of injuries happening—if so, how does that relate to the training presented?

Do workers even remember what was in your training?

Every situation is different, and you will need to define your own success metrics. But doing so up front will help focus your curriculum to the key information and techniques your workers need to stay safe. If what you are presenting cannot be evaluated a month or a year down the line, for the change it produced (not the knowledge it passed on), maybe it's not worth wasting everyone's time.

If you are supervising other trainers, you must absolutely insist on an up-front definition of training success, and how those metrics will be tracked.

MAKE SURE YOU'RE NOT JUST TRACKING CYA OR "TABLE STAKES" TRAINING

For a full discussion of metrics, see chapter nine. But in my golden rules, I have to point out the danger of thinking that "check the box," mandatory training is actually accomplishing anything.

The perfect example is the standard WHMIS, or Workplace Hazardous Material Information System training for workers handling dangerous chemicals and so forth. Yes, WHMIS is required by law. No, it will not be effective without the kind of full training engagement I advocate here.

Keeping stats on things like WHMIS attendance will only satisfy a legal requirement, it won't tell you if you're doing your job.

13. FOLLOW-UP AND REINFORCEMENT TRAINING

Everyone needs reinforcement training. Athletes, musicians, police, you name it. Humans forget things. They get lazy. If they don't do a task for a month, they start to lose their edge.

But somehow, in industrial settings, all the safety training seems to get frontloaded when people join the company—even if it's just a boring video or slideshow.

You absolutely need to repeat topics every few months, to the very same people. Before you do so, of course, you need to do another needs assessment, and you need to talk to those people, to see what's actually happening on the ground—then adjust your presentation.

If you've gotten past mere PowerPoint to a more *interactive, demonstrative training technique,* you won't even have to update any slides.

14. SPEAK ADULT TO ADULT

I've said this five or ten times in different ways, but I'm going to repeat it here because it is so often forgotten by trainers.

You are speaking to adults, not children.

If you say, "Okay guys, we're doing something frigging dangerous here, let's figure out how to protect our hands while we're doing it" people will become engaged.

If you say, "I'm now going to show you the safe way to do this," part of everyone's brain will rebel and tune you out because you are treating them like a child. It's that simple.

How Adults Learn

You must also remember that unlike children, adults learn by relating new information to their existing experience. If you talk about the safe way to hold a welding torch, you will probably be talking to people who have been welding for years.

You always need to start from where they are today, and move on from there. Never from square one.

You have to say, "Jim, show me how you hold your torch" before you adjust the way Jim holds a torch.

Finally, remember that adult learning is not content-oriented, it's problem-oriented. *Adults only gather information to solve problems.* That means you always have to present the problem, and get people to *agree* that it's a problem, before you get to the solution.

IF YOU TRAIN IN NOTHING ELSE...

Using this book, some outside resources (see Appendix 3), and your own experience, I know you can create a great hand-safety training presentation. But if you want to have a serious impact on safety culture, I implore you to present at least these two key ideas:

If workers see something, they must feel free to say something... and be willing to stop the work process if necessary. The history of safety is packed with stories of people who could have said something to stop a horrible accident, but did not. The Korean co-pilot who was too deferential to the pilot to point out that their plane was in imminent danger of crashing.[106]

The 1987 King's Cross Station fire which was at first ignored by staff, who were each operating in their own purview, which did not include dealing with fires. Only passengers seemed to notice and raise alarms. The result was thirty-one dead and dozens injured.[107] The disaster at the Deepwater Horizon platform, where lots of people said nothing when something needed to be said.[108] In training sessions, you must explicitly give workers permission and encouragement to report safety issues, and even call out for work to stop until something is fixed. Say, "This is part of our culture at this company," and make that statement true.

Injuries have long-term, not short-term consequences. Young people are particularly prone to the strange idea that an injury means N days out of work, maybe a surgery, then back on the job. The reality is very different. Hand injuries often mean months of therapy, lost jobs, damaged marriages, and years of cascading consequences. Hand injuries often change lives forever. Ask the minister in the sidebar above. Go back and read more discussion about this terrible truth in chapter one. Formulate challenging statements: Does a training session participant love to fish? One wrong move at the drill press, and maybe they could never fish again.

LOOKING FOR TALENT

Most of the advice in this chapter is aimed at trainers. If you are not a trainer yourself, but oversee trainers, I need to be straight up:

You have a responsibility to go listen to your trainers give their talks, help them to be personable and engaging, and coach them on all this until you see success.

Importantly, however, you must also be willing to change trainers out.

Far too often, managers in industrial settings put up with safety trainers who don't even seem to *like* public speaking, much less study it as an art. Just because someone is good and even safe at performing the actual work, it doesn't mean they're good at talking about it publicly.

Even worse are managers who designate someone to do training who doesn't even want the job—as if safety training were a grim necessity instead of a privilege and a responsibility.

A lot of managers just figure, "If we give this PowerPoint we've checked the safety box, and we can move on. Anyone can give this show. We're presenting the information. Whether or not these guys take it to heart is up to them."

Nothing could be more wrongheaded.

It's even worse when executives just pad the rolls of safety trainers with untrained and untested names in order to meet regulatory quotas. Often they pad the rolls with people like Crissy, who we read about earlier in the sidebar: the woman who got the safety job because she took too long in the restroom, and was late to a meeting.

Safety training requires a broad and rare mix of skills: the ability to engage, to establish credibility, to show empathy, and to introduce some humor. Few people have the whole package. Nevertheless, it's your job as a manager to find and cultivate talented trainers, and never to put up with mediocrity. People's hands are at stake.

I could summarize this chapter as: 1) deeply know the hazards, 2) deeply know your audience, 3) create linkage to larger safety efforts, 4) engage fully, and 5) track meaningfully. Which pieces are you missing in your work?

CHAPTER NINE

GOOD METRICS AND USELESS METRICS

"If you cannot measure it, you cannot improve it."

—LORD KELVIN, 1824-1907

Let's get something straight, right off:

The purpose of keeping hand-safety metrics is not to show how safe workers were in your company over the last year, or the last quarter—or even if they're safe this morning. Metrics must show you; 1) how to save workers' hands in the future, and 2) if you're actually doing those things.

That's the key difference between *lagging indicators* and *leading indicators,* a difference which lies at the heart of this chapter. Lagging indicators show you the past. Leading indicators attempt to show you the future. Blowing a tire is a lagging indicator; the number of regular tire inspections is a leading indicator. Until recent years, most people in dangerous industries did not grasp the difference. They may or may not have known exactly how safe workers were *yesterday*, but they complacently used yesterday's numbers to draw useless conclusions about how safe they would be *tomorrow*.

Take the famous explosion at a BP refinery in Texas City on March 23, 2005 at 1:20 p.m. that killed fifteen workers and injured 180. On the very day of the explosion, indeed right before the explosion, the project coordinator, William Bradley Bessire, held a "safety lunch" to reward workers in his section for the many weeks without an accident—a *lagging* indicator carefully compiled. No doubt ignored during the lunch presentations was an important *leading* indicator: In January of 2005, a consulting firm had found numerous safety issues, including "broken alarms, thinned pipe, chunks of concrete falling, bolts dropping sixty feet (18 m) and staff being overcome with fumes." The report's co-author had stated, "We have never seen a site where the notion 'I could die today' was so real." According to reports in the *Financial Times*, the explosion came shortly after Mr. Bessire finished a big plate of fajitas, rice and beans, congratulated the workers on another good week, and headed back to his office.[109]

THE PROBLEM WITH LAGGING INDICATORS

The number of people who suffered serious injuries last year is certainly an important number to know, and it fulfills your government-reporting requirements. But it tells you absolutely nothing about safety efforts underway, issues building up, or progress made against infrastructure goals. The government-mandated records that BP kept about past injuries certainly told BP nothing about the explosion about to occur.[110]

THE "RECORDABLE RATE" EFFECT

Government reporting mandates are just table stakes. Useful metrics are a tool for you to make your people safer.

In the US, for example, the Occupational Safety and Health Administration (OSHA) has specific requirements for businesses to track injuries and fatalities, with a single number tracking the number of "recordable injuries" per one hundred employees per 200,000 hours worked. This is called the TRIR, which stands for Total Recordable Injuries Rate—an absurdly simple number. Within the TRIR, a fatality counts as one, and a cut that requires two stitches counts as one. Indeed, OSHA says, to paraphrase:

> Recordable work-related injuries and illnesses are those that result in one or more of the following: medical treatment beyond first aid, one or more days away from work, restricted work or transfer to another job, diagnosis of a significant injury or illness, loss of consciousness, or death.[111]

People say, without any context, that a TRIR of 3.0 or less is good, and of course a TRIR of 0.0 is perfect. But the problem with this totally lagging indicator is that companies often view their safety performance through that one number, *which gives no meaningful or actionable detail.* As in, "We've got a great TRIR, so we must be a good, safe company!"

Wrong.

You will need to get way beyond calculating your TRIR if you have any hope of understanding and improving the safety at your company. Certainly you won't be able to improve something as specific as hand safety.

THE REVOLUTION

The ongoing revolution in the way we think about metrics came in no small part from the efforts of Dr. David Michaels, who led OSHA for seven years starting in 2010.

Well before his tenure, Michaels was advocating the use of leading indicators over lagging indicators. While at the agency, he used his bully pulpit to help change minds throughout the industry.[112] Today, the concept of leading indicators is widely accepted as gospel, but not everyone has gotten the message, and the use of leading indicators remains spotty and sometimes clumsy.

In this chapter, I want to give you practical advice on how to retool your own thinking about numbers, and especially hand-safety numbers.

A BRIEF HISTORY OF STATS

The history of safety metrics is not impressive.

In the early days of the Industrial Revolution, nobody tracked injuries, much less compliance with safety standards. Only as labor unions began to demand better conditions, did government organizations respond by putting in regulations and forcing safer conditions for workers.

In the US, each agency and its rules were at first only industry-specific, so there wasn't much consistency—neither in what safety measures were required, nor in what had to be tracked over time. A lot of regulations were driven by disasters—and were, again, industry-focused. For example, the 1907 mine explosion that killed over 360 workers was the impetus for the US Congress to create the US Bureau of Mines.

In 1912, the Bureau of Labor Statistics issued its first annual report on injury rates, but it was focused specifically on the iron and steel industry. The effort was broadened to all industries only in 1926, and the US Occupational Safety and Health Administration (OSHA) wasn't created until 1971, finally bringing genuine consistency not just to US safety efforts, but inspiring efforts worldwide. Nevertheless, in the beginning, OSHA only selected certain companies to report stats, and unreliably extrapolated industry stats from there.

Companies themselves tended to focus only on the cost of injuries.

For a long time, at companies and within governmental agencies, little was reported about the *context and circumstances* of injuries, making it impossible to use the raw numbers to make clear improvements. Only in 1992 did OSHA start collecting at least some more detailed information, including things like days missed from work, and whether employees were later restricted in their work or transferred to a different kind of job because of these injuries.

Shockingly, OSHA was also for a long time seriously tracking only *injuries and fatalities,* not long-term *occupational illnesses*—a much harder task. A 2007 study, for example, estimated there were more than *nine times as many fatal occupational illnesses as there were fatal injuries in the workplace!*[113]

Only in 2015 did OSHA begin requiring employers to report not just fatalities, but severe injuries within twenty-four hours—

hospitalization, amputation, or loss of an eye. In the first year, about 10,000 such injuries were reported, which OSHA believed to be about 50 percent compliance.[114]

Since the time of former Assistant Secretary David Michaels (see above), OSHA has become an important advocate of leading indicators over lagging indicators. In the words of the agency, "...leading indicators are proactive, preventive, and predictive measures that provide information about the effective performance of your safety and health activities. They measure events leading up to injuries, illnesses, and other incidents and reveal potential problems in your safety and health program. In contrast, lagging indicators measure the occurrence and frequency of events that occurred in the past, such as the number or rate of injuries, illnesses, and fatalities."[115]

CREATING LEADING HAND-SAFETY INDICATORS

Once you get onboard the metrics revolution, you need to start identifying leading indicators to aid your own hand-safety program.

Fair warning: this will not be nearly as easy as tracking lagging indicators like injuries, lost days, trips to the ER, or even long-term health effects. Selecting and tracking leading indicators will require careful planning, logical foresight, and well-considered limits on scope.

Suppose you're running a plant in which workers frequently handle caustic chemicals. Instead of merely tracking reported injuries, consider tracking:

- Number of times workers are spotted not wearing gloves

- Number of regular hand-safety training sessions and number of attendees
- Number of workers who can pass a quick test on how to safely don and doff gloves in a hazardous chemical environment
- Number and result of cleanliness inspections per month
- Number and result of pipe joint inspections per quarter
- Number of times an employee exercised their "stop work authority" after spotting an issue. (A high number is a good thing. It means employees feel comfortable and empowered to watch out for one another.)
- Near misses (Once you encourage workers to report them!)
- Employee complaints and safety feedback

In short, as one expert put it, "Leading indicators capture the presence of safety as opposed to the absence of injury."[116]

Each situation will be different—and as always, effective metrics begin with an effective hazard assessment. But well-chosen metrics will tell you if safety is improving or is being neglected—and precisely how you can make improvements. Lagging metrics like recordable injury rates and near-miss rates should back up your analysis.

Each metric should also be linked to a *goal*. Perhaps a goal of zero times per month that a worker is spotted without gloves. Once per month hand-safety training sessions with 90 percent attendance. One hundred percent of workers able to pass the don and doff test. And so forth.

The tools for gathering this kind of information will be varied. The safety manager may do personal inspections, but supervisors must support the effort by themselves becoming observers and recorders of safety issues. Are people wearing their PPE? Are worksites staying clean and orderly? Ideally, workers too would contribute to your stats by faithfully reporting near misses and issues with *absolutely no fear of retribution or penalties to their coworkers.*

Experts call your overall strategy for gathering safety data your *surveillance system*, a somewhat unfriendly phrase for a vital part of your organization.

BREAKING DOWN THE KINDS OF INDICATORS

The Campbell Institute at the National Safety Council has published a helpful whitepaper[117] on creating leading indicators and safety surveillance systems. They found it useful to break the indicators into three major categories:

- *Operations-based leading indicators:* infrastructure, machinery, maintenance. These may be site-specific.
- *Systems-based leading indicators:* Indicators that relate to the administration and management of safety: training, monitoring, staffing, forward planning. These can be rolled up from a facility level to a region/business unit or corporate level.
- *Behavior-based leading indicators:* Indicators that measure the behavior or actions of individuals or groups in the workplace. Are people wearing their PPE? Reporting concerns? Following protocol on the job?

See Appendix 6 for links to case studies and more ideas on creating leading indicator metrics.

CONTEXT IS EVERYTHING

Once you start shifting your mindset on metrics, you will also realize that *context* matters as much or more than numbers, especially in injury reporting.

If someone burnt their hand with a caustic chemical, why did that happen? Was the shop unclean? Were the tops of the chemical containers loose due to worn threading? Were the wrong gloves worn? Is something missing in your hazard assessments?

Only with that kind of information can you respond to make the environment safer, and to shift the focus of your leading indicators. How often are containers inspected and replaced? Are all workers trained on the right gloves for different kinds of caustics? Are cleanliness inspections occurring on schedule?

No context? Your numbers are simply useless. I remember one time our team was called in to a large auto assembly factory to help reduce their hand injuries. When we asked for their data, they said, "We had sixty hand injuries last year!" When we asked for details by department and injury type, they just looked at us blankly. "Oh, we don't have that information." We stared back, not sure what to do next. Were all those injuries at a single point in the line, maybe where workers fasten on the axles? No one knew.

Valuable context can only be gathered from the people closest to the event. Once again, that means all workers must understand and be involved positively in your monitoring efforts—not isolated from the reporting process.

Include a searchable narrative text field in every electronic injury report. You never know what future trends may be identified from analysis of these fields. Is the word "turbine" recurring, over and over in accident reports? Maybe somebody should look at those turbines.

MANAGING THE SCOPE OF INDICATORS

The right safety data collection may be invaluable, but it is certainly possible to have too much of a good thing. Once you start down the road of leading indicators, you can see how the sheer number of variables could lead to over-bureaucratization and over-gathering of information.

Limits on leading indicators are tough to determine, but vital to create.

Carefully choose what to measure so you do not overburden your staff and the greater organization. Measuring requires time, effort, and money; if you're measuring the wrong thing, it can be a huge problem, and it can undercut or destroy your organizational support for monitoring.

Over-gathering can also lead to misleading shortcuts. For example, if you demand 300 different codes for injuries, people will stop paying attention to your codes, and just use two or three of their favorites. Pick the right ten codes, and your data may actually be more accurate.[118]

I'll be honest here: the balance between the *specificity* and *efficiency* of your surveillance system will be hard to achieve, and will require lots of conversation. But over time, experience and refinement will show useful results—and create a safety legacy that can be passed to future generations at your company.

USING "NATURAL EXPERIMENTS"

One great way to gather useful data without needless bureaucracy is to look for what I'll call "natural experiments" already occurring within your company or your industry, in which a change is made at one site while the same change has not been made (or not yet been made) at another site.

For example, suppose a hand-safety training program is rolled out in Pittsburgh, but not yet in Scranton. Is there a relative change in injury rates? Safety morale? If data gathering *is identical or at least similar at both sites,* useful knowledge about the program's effectiveness might be gained painlessly. The same can be true of different equipment used at different sites, and so forth.

Where can you see natural experiments occurring within your organization? Do you have consistent enough monitoring to use the resulting data effectively?

USING UNIVERSAL LEADING INDICATORS

While many of your leading indicators will be highly specific to your company, some are universal. For example, experts have identified "Four Safety Truths" that everyone should track:[119]

- *Safety Truth #1: More inspections predict a safer worksite. So you should set goals, and track your numbers of inspections.*
- *Safety Truth #2: More inspectors, specifically more inspectors outside the safety function, predict a safer worksite. So you should track the number and variety of inspectors. More inspector types = fewer cognitive biases.*
- *Safety Truth #3: Too many "100 percent safe" inspections predict an unsafe worksite. Unless you track these, you won't hear the alarm bell that your inspectors aren't doing their job.*
- *Safety Truth #4: Too many unsafe observations predict an unsafe worksite. Obviously, right? But do you know how many unsafe observations were made in your company last month?*

Each of these stats could be tracked as say, a three-month moving average against each 50,000 hours of work.

MONITORING THE RESULTS OF SAFETY INITIATIVES

One of the most important functions of metrics is to find out if your safety initiatives and programs are making a difference. As I said, every initiative needs to be launched with a set of key indicators that can be tracked before and after.

Indeed, it's entirely possible that a program will have a negative effect—alienating workers, or introducing unexpectedly dangerous changes to technique. In one case, a Ford assembly plant started a fitness program to reduce back injuries among its employees. Six months out, the lost-day rate from back injuries had gone up from fourteen to twenty-two cases. Long-term muscular problems doubled.

Without good metrics, no one would have known to shut the program down.[120]

THE EFFECTIVENESS ISSUE

Measuring effectiveness, of course, comes with a load of difficulties.

Suppose you were seeing a hand-pinching rate with a tire-balancing machine of one injury per quarter. A year into a specific hand-safety training program, that number went to zero. Is this change statistically significant? After all, incident rates can fluctuate without any change in behavior at all.

Or suppose your company has an OSHA recordable injury rate of 1.75. You start a safety program and a year later, your rate is still 1.75. It doesn't mean that you've made no progress, because you can't measure what you have prevented.

A better measure might be to poll workers before and after the program, to see what number feels safer, and if they feel that new safety techniques are helping. With some careful thought, you will find a leading indicator to measure your success. If you've spent a lot of money on this safety program, you might well need such stats to prove to your board that their money was well spent.

Of course, you should also monitor a program's results on an ongoing basis, so you can make changes and adjustments as it's happening. You shouldn't have to wait six months, like at that Ford plant, to see if you are inadvertently harming people's backs.

PREVENTING OVERREACTION TO INDIVIDUAL INCIDENTS

One of the biggest benefits of tracking leading indicators is to refocus attention from the short to the long-term. Indeed, one of the most important reasons to carefully investigate and track the context of injuries is to determine if accidents, or even strings of accidents, are freak occurrences, or if they indicate a systematic issue.

It's far too common for a tragic, but outlying accident or series of accidents to divert attention and resources from ongoing safety programs. This is a case of lagging indicators trumping leading indicators, to the detriment of safety.

In one of his excellent books, safety expert, Thomas Krause, tells a revealing story about just such a case:

> So we once worked on a safety improvement project with a refinery in Louisiana. The effort was driven by a steering committee comprised of front line employees, requiring little from

site management, except allocation of time to the workers. Over a period of two years, the steering committee developed a first rate safety improvement process, engaging workers and getting results. Awareness was high, behaviors were improving, and teams were finding work reconfiguration projects and executing them well. So safety numbers were coming down consistently, and they were statistically significant. It was a model project.

Then over a two month period, they had a number of incidents, seemingly out of the blue. The steering committee tested for statistical significance and concluded the incidents were due to normal variations. They looked at leading indicators and found no basis for alarm or redirection of their efforts. The best decision they could make was to stay the course.

But a new plant manager saw the increased numbers and pushed the panic button. It looked to him like the program that he was taking credit for was suddenly faltering. In truth, he knew virtually nothing about the program and his relationship to safety was no more sophisticated than looking at the endpoint numbers [in other words, the lagging indicators].

...He made the decision—without consulting with the steering committee—that the number of safety observations must go up, and the way he would ensure [more safety observations] was to tie an observational goal to a financial incentive. He thought he was taking the action needed to address a problem decisively. But he was actually destroying the hard work and spent resources of two years of work.[121]

It is vital to remember, says Krause, that "leading indicators and longitudinal root cause analysis give a more complete picture of workplace safety than incident numbers. We can't rely on outcome data alone to tell us about the safety of the workplace. You could cut [risk exposure] by 30 percent in a quarter and your injury rate may still go up. You could let exposure creep up by 10 or 15 percent in a quarter, and your injury rate could go down. Injuries and exposure never track perfectly."[122]

In other words, don't overreact to individual events. Gather the right long-term data and take a long-term view. Basic good management, right? But often not applied to safety, where panicky "pinball" safety measures, bouncing from incident to incident, may rule management's thinking.

THE SAFETY CULTURE BENEFITS OF LEADING INDICATORS

Another important benefit of leading indicators is a focus on the positive.

When safety is discussed only in reaction to an accident, it becomes linked to negative consequences in the minds of everyone, and a positive culture of safety never develops. After an incident, those CEO memos sent companywide with "thoughts and prayers," along with their dark reminders to observe safety rules, serve only to make *safety* a grim word in the company vocabulary.

Leading indicators help create the positive team spirit and responsibility necessary for a strong safety culture within a company: "Yes, we're doing training! Yes, people are wearing their gloves! Yes, we got those gears caged on the shredder!"

BE VERY PUBLIC ABOUT INDICATORS

To build your safety culture, however, both the indicators and the resulting data must be shared with everyone—instead of hidden away in management meetings. Highly public leading indicators help people get past their cognitive biases, look for things to fix, and take proactive steps together.

Indeed, without the tracking of leading indicators, people at all levels will tend to ignore existing risk factors because an accident "hasn't happened yet."

In short, according to safety expert, Aubrey Daniels,[123] leading indicators:

- Allow you to see and celebrate small improvements
- Make it clear what actually needs to be done to get better
- Encourage constructive problem-solving
- Measure the positive: what people are doing, instead of failing to do
- Enable frequent feedback to all stakeholders—not just when injuries occur
- Build credibility for a safety program
- Track impact versus intention

You can pop those bullet points right into your PowerPoint to your management team, justifying the money you want to spend on data gathering.

COMPANIONS FOR YOUR JOURNEY

One final note to help you rethink your stats.

Searching for the right stats is like looking for the right companions to take on a long and dangerous journey. They will influence you, and you will influence them as you move forward.

Take the right stats on your journey, and like good friends, they will prompt you to *take* action, take the *right* actions, and keep those actions in the proper *priority*.

Take the right stats along, and through their positive influence, they will also help you win more friends and companions in your quest. By tracking the leading indicators which show "progress in our safety," you are not just fulfilling the highest goals of your work, you are getting everyone onboard.

And of course, only when everyone is finally onboard will the journey become safe.

CONCLUSION

IN THE END, IT'S ALL PERSONAL

I started this book talking about the three kinds of companies I visit in the course of my work selling gloves. Companies that do a good job on safety. Companies that do a terrible job. Companies trying to do better.

But as I reach the end, it's not the companies I remember. Not the boardrooms. Not the purchasing managers. It's the faces of people I've met scattered out on crowded shop floors. Strung along high-speed production lines. That guy handling steel rods up on a scaffolding. That gal running ore into a smelting vat.

People with lovers to touch. Children to hold. Parents to embrace.

I ask, "What am I doing to keep these people safe?" I ask, "What are you doing?"

Because in the end, it's all personal.

A CEO like Paul O'Neill of Alcoa stands up at a management meeting and announces that he and all his staff are personally responsible for the death of a young worker.

A VP like David White of Campbell's Soup makes a personal phone call to the immediate supervisor of an injured employee, anywhere in the world, every single time a serious report comes in.

Before he begins his hand-safety talk, a trainer tells a personal story to show he's seen tragedies up close.

A supervisor encourages a worker to stand up and share her personal tales of near misses on the line.

To paraphrase safety expert, Danielle Kretschmer, the personal happens when one worker leans over to another and says, "Hey, dude. You know, we go barbeque together. We go to church together. Our kids play together. Put your PPE on."[124]

IT ONLY TAKES ONE PERSON

Do you have the leverage to make change happen?

Maybe you're not a CEO or a VP. Maybe those people don't even know your name. But safe practices, like unsafe practices, propagate virally. There are dozens of stories of improvements made at far-flung sites that ultimately changed the practices of multinational companies. Dozens of stories of single safety managers, way down the org chart, who shifted a culture forever.

Sometimes it only takes one person who gets it. One person who talks the talk and walks the walk.

One person who recognizes that small changes add up.

IT ONLY TAKES A HUNDRED LITTLE ACTIONS

I love the story of David Brailsford, the British cycling coach, who decided to improve his team's performance not with some groundbreaking new technique, but with an aggregation of tiny improvements.[125]

Brailsford inspired his team to get one percent better at every single thing they did, until the gains added up. They slept on better beds for more hours of the night. They avoided shaking hands at competitions so they wouldn't pick up germs. He looked at anything and everything for a little marginal edge. And it worked. They performed better. They started winning gold. Dominating world championships.

Rethinking hand safety is a lot like that. It's never one action, it's a hundred actions, repeated again and again.

It's corporate discipline. It's forward planning. It's psychology. It's culture. It's infrastructure. It's administration. It's behavior modification. It's training. It's keeping the right stats.

And always, it's about taking it personally. Always, it's about you looking someone else in the eye and saying, "We're going to do these hundred things together."

THE MULTIPLIER EFFECT

If ever you feel discouraged, don't forget that you have the multiplier effect on your side.

I guarantee that doing a hundred apparently insignificant things will have a far bigger impact than you first observe.

If you make a small improvement in the safety of a line, an employee may go away saying to himself, "Okay, this person cares about me and has my back." That employee will talk to others. Others will talk to others. People will start looking for more improvements. They'll listen the next time you speak. Eventually they'll try out those better gloves you recommend.

Give it time.

JOINING THE TRIBE

Finally, part of getting personal is joining the tribe.

It's pretty rare for managers, especially upper managers, to have a tribe. You find a lot of false bonhomie on a thirtieth floor. Some drinking, maybe some mutual admiration, but rarely a genuine "I have your back, you have my back" kind of brotherhood or sisterhood. There's rarely a genuine "We're in this together, buddy" feeling in a glass conference room.

Among people who work with their hands, however, tribalism is vital and tribalism is real. Workers really do cover for each other, watch each other's backs, sacrifice for one another. They don't care much about looks or education or the ability to speak well. They care about proven skills, meaningful experience, human authenticity, and personal loyalty.

Especially loyalty.

It's really hard for upper managers to grasp what this means. Even harder to join in.

When upper managers come down to talk on a shop floor, workers sometimes call it a "beauty pageant." The managers show off their suits, their vocabulary, their smarts. Just like Miss America, they do the wave, they do a turn on the catwalk, then they're gone. No one much listens to what they say, because no one believes they mean it.

In a true culture of safety, however, managers really do become part of the working tribe. Everyone really does feel like they're in it together.

Easier said than done? It takes persistence and special tactics, but it's completely possible. Take a cue from Charles Piper, EHS manager at Exide Technologies, a plastic manufacturing facility:

> [When I started, I went to a manager and I said] I wanted to spend a week doing production work, because it's one thing for me to stand there and watch somebody load a press and unload a press, and trim cases and stack them. It's quite another to actually do it. He looked at me like I'd grown two heads. We went to our shift supervisors and I said, "Okay, I'm going to be working on first shift for these 3 days and I'm going to work third shift these 2 days. Put me at the heaviest places." They think, "okay." For a week, I was out there and people were laughing at first, and then they were like, "Oh, you're serious about doing this." One, I think that gave them a little bit of eye-opening…"Here's a manager who's willing to get his hands dirty and get out here, instead of standing here and telling us what to do," and it gives me a firsthand look at what they do.[126]

Over time, Piper and his workers felt like they were in it together.

If you demonstrate a real concern for safety, if you get your hands dirty, and if you ask, "How can I make this easier for you, safer for you, better for you?" and then you actually follow through—eventually you will break in.

Again, give it time. It takes a hell of a lot of work to make people believe you're not just in it for the money, or to put on a show. But at some point a tipping point will come when people start seeing that the words you say and the actions you take are meaningful and authentic.

When that happens, the magic of personal connection will happen, too.

You will be part of the tribe. Body and soul.

MY CHARGE TO YOU

As you finish this book, I ask you to raise a hand up to your eyes. Turn it slowly and marvel again at its beauty, its ingenuity, its balance, its intelligence, its tenacity—its fragility.

Whether you are a CEO, a supervisor, or a safety manager, I ask you to recognize that it's not just about statistics, or the big picture, or accountability.

It's about human hands.

It's about all those workers going home to their families each night, fully intact: able to caress their spouse's face, tousle their children's hair.

I guarantee that nothing in your life will be more satisfying than seeing injuries go down because of your tiniest and most incremental of efforts: a safety guard added to a machine, the right kind of gloves actually used, a light dawning on a worker's face during a talk you give.

I guarantee that your journey of small improvements will have a visible and profound impact on the lives of others.

I ask you to take this charge personally.

Go out and save some hands.

APPENDICES AND SUPPORTING WEBSITE

I urge you to check out the supporting website for this book, at www.rethinkinghandsafety.com. There you will find a huge number of resources, including the specific materials referenced in the appendices below.

Especially be sure to check out the Hand Safety Culture Quiz and the Hand Safety Checklist.

APPENDIX 1: GLOVE SELECTION REFERENCES
1A: CHOOSING THE RIGHT CUT LEVEL

www.superiorglove.com/en/work-gloves-101/
guide-to-choosing-the-right-cut-resistant-gloves.

www.superiorglove.com/blog/wp-content/uploads/Superior-Glove-
Choosing-The-Right-Cut-Resistant-Glove2.pdf.

1B: TWO KINDS OF PUNCTURE THREATS

www.superiorglove.com/en/work-gloves-101/
guide-to-choosing-the-best-puncture-resistant-gloves.

1C: LEATHER GLOVE CONSIDERATIONS

www.superiorglove.com/en/work-gloves-101/
guide-to-selecting-a-leather-work-glove.

1D: A SHORT GUIDE TO GLOVE COATINGS

www.superiorglove.com/blog/guide-for-palm-coated-work-gloves.

www.superiorglove.com/blog/battle-of-the-palm-coatings.

1E: SLEEVES AND LONG CUFFS

https://www.superiorglove.com/blog/
how-to-choose-the-right-cut-resistant-sleeves.

1F: TYPICAL GLOVE MATERIALS

www.superiorglove.com/blog/dyneema-vs-kevlar.

1G: LINKS TO GLOVE CHOOSING TOOLS

www.superiorglove.com/en/glove-selector.

1H: GLOVE LAUNDERING RECOMMENDATIONS

www.superiorglove.com/blog/
are-you-throwing-money-out-with-your-dirty-gloves.

1I: IMPACT RESISTANCE STANDARDS

www.superiorglove.com/blog/everything-you-need-to-know-about-ansi-isea-138-the-new-impact-standard.

1J: ANTI-VIBRATION GLOVE INFORMATION

As I noted in the text, for tools with high levels of vibration, like a jackhammer, choose a glove with a lot of anti-vibration padding, for smaller tools like a grinder, go with a thinner, more form-fitting glove. A glove with too much padding can actually increase forearm strain and increase the likelihood of HAVS.

Here's a glove with lots of padding: https://www.superiorglove.com/en/vibrastop-anti-vibration-full-finger-gloves.

Here's a more form-fitting antivibe glove: https://www.superiorglove.com/en/goatskin-leather-palm-full-finger-vibration-dampening-gloves.

APPENDIX 2: SAMPLE GLOVE EVALUATION
2A: NEW GLOVE EVALUATION FORM

https://rethinkinghandsafety.com/hand-safety-resources/.

2B: SAMPLE GLOVE TRIAL SURVEY

https://rethinkinghandsafety.com/hand-safety-resources/.

APPENDIX 3: HAZARD ASSESSMENT RESOURCES
3A: HAND HAZARD TRACKING SPREADSHEET

https://rethinkinghandsafety.com/hand-safety-resources/.

3B: HAND HAZARD ASSESSMENT QUESTIONS CHECKLIST

https://rethinkinghandsafety.com/hand-safety-resources/.

3C: THIRD-PARTY HAND HAZARD ASSESSMENT RESOURCES

https://www.dsslearning.com/hand-safety-it-s-in-your-hands/ HAN002/.

https://www.training.dupont.com/ pause-for-performance-hand-safety/MLPP01/.

https://www.convergencetraining.com.

https://www.americantrainingresources.com/spv-38.aspxcom/ hand-safety.html.

http://www.intertek.com/high-risk-industry/ hand-injury-prevention-training/.

APPENDIX 4: MINDFULNESS RESOURCES

https://www.theglobeandmail.com/report-on-business/careers/workplace-award/ how-mindfulness-improved-nb-powers-safety-record/ article38239933/.

https://www.rmsswitzerland.com/assets/mindful-safety.pdf.

www.headspace.com.

APPENDIX 5: TRAINING RESOURCES

https://rethinkinghandsafety.com/hand-safety-resources/.

APPENDIX 6: HAND SAFETY CHECKLIST

I urge you to download and make good use of the spreadsheet at https://rethinkinghandsafety.com/hand-safety-resources/, which includes a checklist for creating your own hand-safety plan. It's partly based on this book, and can easily be modified for your particular company.

APPENDIX 7: ROI CALCULATORS

Need to demonstrate the ROI of safety and glove purchases?

See my company's website at https://www.superiorglove.com/en/roi-calculator.

OSHA in the US provides one at https://www.osha.gov/dcsp/smallbusiness/safetypays/estimator.html.

Another good one can be found at the Queensland Government site in Australia: https://www.worksafe.qld.gov.au/forms-and-resources/tools/workplace-health-and-safety-queensland/return-on-investment-calculator.

NOTES

1   My father, Frank Geng, who was raised in Hungary and Germany tanning leather for gloves, emigrated to Canada after WWII and bought Superior Glove (then Acton Glove) in 1962. It had been in business since 1910. My brother Tony serves as the current president of Superior Glove, and I serve as VP. You can learn more about the company at https://www.superiorglove.com/en/about-us.

2   Majestic Glove, "Workplace Hand Injury Research Study: Findings and Analysis," Last modified September 8, 2016, http://www.majesticglove.com/media/resources/Majestic_Hand%20Injury%20Whitepaper.pdf.

3   "Hands-On Advice to Protect Your Hands," National Safety Council, last modified January 27, 2014, http://www.nsc.org/Membership%20Site%20Document%20Library/Safety-Talks/Safety-Talks-Hand-Protection.pdf.

4   Majestic Glove, "Workplace Hand Injury Research Study: Findings and Analysis." Last modified September 8, 2016, http://www.majesticglove.com/media/resources/Majestic_Hand%20Injury%20Whitepaper.pdf.

5   "Type of Injury or Illness and Body Parts Affected by Nonfatal Injuries and Illnesses in 2014," U.S. Bureau of Labor Statistics, last modified December 2, 2015, https://www.bls.gov/opub/ted/2015/type-of-injury-or-illness-and-body-parts-affected-by-nonfatal-injuries-and-illnesses-in-2014.htm.

6   American Society of Safety Engineers, "White Paper Addressing the Return on Investment for Safety, Health, and Environmental (SH&E) Management Programs," last modified June 8, 2002, http://elcosh.org/document/1082/d000047/asse-white-paper-addressing-the-return-on-investment-for-safety,-health-and-environmental-(sh%26e)-management-programs.html.

7 According to the Executive Survey of Workplace Safety by the Liberty Mutual Group, the leading US provider of worker's compensation insurance, 95 percent of executives report that workplace safety has a positive impact on a company's financial performance. Of those executives, 61 percent believe their companies receive a return on investment of $3 or more for each $1 invested in improving workplace safety. Liberty Mutual, "A Majority of US Businesses Report Workplace Safety Delivers a Return on Investment," Liberty Mutual News Release, Boston, August 28, 2001, http://www.libertymutual.com.

8 Michelle Chen, "Amputated Hands and Torn Fingers: The Meat-Processing Industry's Horrifying Injuries," *The Nation*, last modified February 24, 2016. https://www.thenation.com/article/amputated-hands-and-torn-fingers-the-meat-processing-industrys-horrifying-injuries/.

9 "What are Your Body Parts Worth?" *Insure.com*, December 10, 2015, https://www.insure.com/life-insurance/body-parts.html.

10 Matthew Hallowell (professor, University of Colorado Boulder), in discussion with interviewer, July 6, 2018.

11 Chen, "Amputated Hands and Torn Fingers."

12 *Ibid.*

13 Guy Quenneville, "Saskatoon's Shercom Industries Fined $420K 3 Years After Teen Died on Work Site," *CBC News*, January 11, 2018, https://www.cbc.ca/news/canada/saskatoon/saskatoon-tire-recycler-fined-18-year-old-died-worksite-1.4482714.

14 "OSHA fines factory owner $570,000 for amputation injury," Morgan & Justice Co. LPA, last modified May 9, 2017, https://www.morganandjustice.com/blog/2017/05/osha-fines-factory-owner-570000-for-amputation-injury.shtml.

15 Steve Patterson (hand protection specialist, Superior Glove), in discussion with interviewer, September 12, 2018.

16 Sam Cunard (Occupational Health and Safety Environmental Compliance Manager, HotWire), in discussion with interviewer, November 12, 2018.

17 Charter Partners, "Paul O'Neill CEO of Alcoa - It's all about safety," YouTube video, June 12, 2015, https://www.youtube.com/watch?v=tC2ucDs_XJY.

18 O'Neill's colleague was Bill O'Rourke, former vice president of sustainability and environment, when O'Neill was there. Carnegie Council for Ethics in International Affairs, "The Power of Safety: How Safe Habits Triggered Responsibility at Alcoa," https://www.carnegiecouncil.org/studio/multimedia/20120905-the-power-of-safety-how-safe-habits-triggered-responsibility-at-alcoa, September 5, 2012.

19 "Within a year of O'Neill's speech, Alcoa's profits would hit a record high. By the time he retired in 2000, the company's annual net income was five times larger than before he arrived, and its market capitalization had risen by $27 billion. Someone who invested a million dollars in Alcoa on the day O'Neill was hired would have earned another million dollars in dividends while he headed the company and the value of their stock would be 5 times bigger when he left. "What's more, all that growth occurred while Alcoa became one of the safest companies in the world. Before O'Neill's arrival, almost every Alcoa plant had at least one accident per week. Once his safety plan was implemented, some facilities would go years without a single employee losing a workday due to an accident. The company's worker injury rate fell to one-twentieth the US average." Charles Duhigg, *The Power of Habit: Why We Do What We Do and How to Change It* (New York: Random House, 2012).

20 The lost workday rate is an OSHA formula that refers to those who are so hurt they can't come back to work. The denominator is 200,000 man-hours (the equivalent of 100 people working a year). So a lost workday rate of 1.86 means that almost two people out of every 100 are getting hurt so bad that they can't come back to work the next day.

21 Tom Krause, "Developing High-Performance Cultures: Why Not Start with Safety?" *ISHN Industrial Safety & Hygiene News,* August 22, 2016, https://www.ishn.com/blogs/16-thought-leadership/post/104629-developing-high-performance-cultures-why-not-start-with-safety.

22 John Mendeloff, et al., *Small Businesses and Workplace Fatality Risk: An Exploratory Analysis* (Santa Monica, CA: RAND Corporation, 2006), https://www.rand.org/pubs/technical_reports/TR371.html. Note, however that small companies are often safer than small "establishments" of a larger company, perhaps because of the presence of an owner onsite.

23 Hester J. Lipscomb, James Nolan, Dennis Patterson, Vince Sticca, and Douglas J. Myers, "Safety, Incentives, and the Reporting of Work-Related Injuries Among Union Carpenters: "You're Pretty Much Screwed if You Get Hurt at Work" *American Journal of Industrial Medicine* 56, no. 4 (2013): 389-399, https://onlinelibrary.wiley.com/doi/full/10.1002/ajim.22128.

24 James McGlothlin, Bryan Hubbard, Fereydoun Aghazadeh, and Sarah Hubbard, "Ergonomics Case Study: Safety Training Issues for Hispanic Construction Workers," *Journal of Occupational and Environmental Hygiene* 6, no. 9 (2009): D45-D50, https://oeh.tandfonline.com/doi/abs/10.1080/15459620903106689?journalCode=uoeh20.

25 Researchers conclude that the relatively high safety risks of migrants can be explained by the background of the migrants on the one hand (e.g., language comprehension, knowledge and understanding of local habits and risk perception), and their working environment on the other hand (temporary work, unskilled and risky work). When it comes to migrants' characteristics, different characteristics are mentioned, such as obedience (e.g., more reluctant to address safety issues), eagerness to earn money quickly, risk perception, language problems, understanding the importance of obeying safety regulations, and unfamiliarity with local standards. Annick Starren, Jos Hornikx, and Kyra Luijters, "Occupational Safety in Multicultural Teams and Organizations: A Research Agenda." *Safety Science* 52 (2013): 43-49, https://www.rug.nl/research/portal/files/19506303/Starren_Hornikx_Luijters_2012.pdf.

26 Thomas A. Arcury, Sara A. Quandt, Altha J. Cravey, Rebecca C. Elmore, and Gregory B. Russell, "Farmworker Reports of Pesticide Safety and Sanitation in the Work Environment," *American Journal of Industrial Medicine* 39, (2001): 487-498, http://citeseerx.ist.psu.edu/viewdoc/download?doi=10.1.1.458.7662&rep=rep1&type=pdf.

27 Xiuwen Sue Dong, Yurong Men, and Knut Ringen, "Work-Related Injuries Among Hispanic Construction Workers—Evidence from the Medical Expenditure Panel Survey," *American Journal of Industrial Medicine* 53, no. 6 (2010): 561-569, https://onlinelibrary.wiley.com/doi/full/10.1002/ajim.20799.

28 3M, *3M Personal Protective Equipment Report* (2009).

29 Steve Roberts (Senior Partner, Safety Performance Solutions, Inc.), in discussion with interviewer, June 28, 2018.

30 A much fuller discussion of cognitive bias can be found in Daniel Kahneman, *Thinking, Fast and Slow* (New York: Farrar, Straus and Giroux, 2011).

31 Ola Svenson, "Are We All Less Risky and More Skillful than Our Fellow Drivers?" *Acta Psychologica* 47, no. 2 (1981): 143–48, doi:10.1016/0001-6918(81)90005-6.

32 Scott Plous, *McGraw-Hill Series in Social Psychology, The Psychology of Judgment and Decision Making* (New York, NY: McGraw-Hill Book Company, 1993).

33 Thomas R. Krause and Kristen J. Bell, *7 Insights Into Safety Leadership*. Safety Leadership Institute: 2015.

34 I. A. Walker, S. Reshamwalla, and I. H. Wilson, "Surgical Safety Checklists: Do They Improve Outcomes?" *BJA: British Journal of Anaesthesia* 109, no. 1 (July 2012): 47–54, https://doi.org/10.1093/bja/aes175.

35 See above, *Small Businesses and Workplace Fatality Risk: An Exploratory Analysis* (Santa Monica, CA: RAND Corporation, 2006)

36 J. M. Greene-Blose, "Deepwater Horizon: Lessons in Probabilities," paper presented at *PMI® Global Congress 2015—EMEA, London, England* (Newtown Square, PA: Project Management Institute, 2015).

37 Duncan Kerr, "Rethinking Safety Performance Metrics in the Utility Industry," *The Engine Room*, 2017, https://www.theengineroom.ca/wp-content/uploads/2017/11/Rethinking-Safety-Performance-Metrics-in-the-Utility-Industry.pdf.

38 Carmen Canfora and Angelika Ottmann. "Of Ostriches, Pyramids, and Swiss Cheese: Risks in Safety-Critical Translations," *Translation Spaces* 7, no. 2 (Nov 2018): 167—201, https://doi.org/10.1075/ts.18002.can

39 S. Adam Brasel and James Gips, "Media Multitasking Behavior: Concurrent Television and Computer Usage," *Cyberpsychology, Behavior, and Social Networking* 14, no. 9 (2011): 527-534, https://www.liebertpub.com/doi/pdfplus/10.1089/cyber.2010.0350.

40 Mark O'Rourke, "Increasing Engagement with Vocational Education and Training: a Case Study of Computer Games-Based Safety Training." *2013 Postgraduate Research Papers: A Compendium* (2013): 113-133. http://library.bsl.org.au/jspui/bitstream/1/4639/1/GriffinT_2013-postgraduate-research-papers-compendium_NCVER-2014.pdf#page=115. See also: Brian Magerko, R. E. Wray, Lisa Holt, and Brian Stensrud, "Improving Interactive Training Through Individualized Content and Increased Engagement," In *The Interservice/Industry Training, Simulation & Education Conference* (I/ITSEC), 2005, pp. 1-11, http://homes.lmc.gatech.edu/~bmagerko6/papers/IITSEC-ISAT-2005.final.pdf.

41 Atsunori Ariga and Alejandro Lleras, "Brief and Rare Mental "Breaks" Keep You Focused: Deactivation and Reactivation of Task Goals Preempt Vigilance Decrements," *Cognition* 118, no. 3 (2011): 439-443, https://doi.org/10.1016/j.cognition.2010.12.007.

42 David A.Lombardi, Gary S. Sorock, Russ Hauser, Philip C. Nasca, Ellen A. Eisen, Robert F. Herrick, and Murray A. Mittleman, "Temporal Factors and the Prevalence of Transient Exposures at the Time of an Occupational Traumatic Hand Injury," *Journal of Occupational and Environmental Medicine* 45, no. 8 (2003): 832-840, https://journals.lww.com/joem/Abstract/2003/08000/Temporal_Factors_and_the_Prevalence_of_Transient.8.aspx.

43 "Night and Evening Shifts Linked to Higher Risk of Injuries: Study," *At Work*, 73, (Summer 2013), *Institute for Work & Health*, https://www.iwh.on.ca/newsletters/at-work/73/night-and-evening-shifts-linked-to-higher-risk-of-injuries-study.

44 A study investigated the link between meditation, self-reported mindfulness and ability to pay attention. It compared a group of meditators experienced in mindfulness meditation with a control group that did not have meditation experience and found that meditators performed significantly better than non-meditators on all measures of attention including mindfulness. Adam Moore and Peter Malinowski, "Meditation, Mindfulness and Cognitive Flexibility," *Consciousness and Cognition* 18, no. 1 (2009): 176-186, https://pdfs.semanticscholar.org/9c9d/4c2564a4529180dd0574a3f3c2e5ecf9617c.pdf.

45 Marissa Afton (Client Solutions Director, The Potential Project), in discussion with interviewer, March 24, 2019.

46 See Kim Witte, "Putting the Fear Back into Fear Appeals: The Extended Parallel Process Model," *Communication Monographs* 59 no. 4 (1992):329-349.

47 Matthew Hallowell, "Live Safety Demonstrations (Full Video)," Vimeo, posted 2017, https://vimeo.com/228901665.

48 William G Shadel, Steven C Martino, Claude M Setodji, Michael Dunbar, Deborah Scharf, Kasey G Creswell, "Do graphic health warning labels on cigarette packages deter purchases at point-of-sale? An experiment with adult smokers," *Health Education Research* 34, No. 3 (June 2019), Pages 321–331, https://academic.oup.com/her/article/34/3/321/5424102.

49 Stephen J. Dubner and Steven D. Levitt, "Selling Soap," *New York Times Magazine*, September 24, 2006, https://www.nytimes.com/2006/09/24/magazine/24wwln_freak.html.

50   S.S. David and K. Goel. "Knowledge, Attitude, and Practice of Sugarcane Crushers Towards Hand Injury Prevention Strategies in India," *Injury Prevention* 7, no. 4 (2001): 329-330, http://injuryprevention.bmj.com/content/7/4/329.

51   Emad A. Gashgari, "Generational Differences in Safety Attitudes Among Commercial Airline Pilots," PhD diss., *Arizona State University*, 2013, https://repository.asu.edu/attachments/110696/content/Gashgari_asu_0010N_13108.pdf.

52   Younger workers are indeed more likely to be injured at work. The correlation is much stronger between time on job (tenure) and injury rate. If you've been in a job for less than 6 months you are 2.5x more likely to be injured than someone on the job for more than 6 months. The takeaway is to do a really good job training new employees. Also, a practical tactic is to have new employees wear a different color uniform or sleeve for a given period of time so they can be easily identified, and other people can easily help them if needed. For example, in some plants, Toyota has new employees wear red arm bands. See "Analysis of the Impact of Job Tenure on Workplace Injury Rates," *Health and Safety Executive*, accessed September 9, 2019, http://www.hse.gov.uk/statistics/adhoc-analysis/workplace-injury-rates.htm.

53   Edward P. Grzybowski Jr, "Behavior Based Safety and the Multi-Generational Workforce," *Eastern Kentucky University*, 2015, https://encompass.eku.edu/cgi/viewcontent.cgi?article=1369&context=etd.

54   Overall, men are more likely to take risks in general. A study comparing male and female workers found differences related to risk of various types of injuries. Male workers were two to four times more likely to report exposure to dust and chemical substances, loud noise, irregular hours, night shifts, and vibrating tools. Women were 30 percent more likely to report repetitive tasks and working at high speed and more likely to report exposure to disinfectants, hair dyes, and textile dust. But when men were compared with women with the same job title, there was not a significant difference between the genders. See James P. Byrnes, David C. Miller, and William D. Schafer, "Gender Differences in Risk Taking: A Meta-Analysis," *Psychological Bulletin* 125, no. 3 (1999): 367, DOI: 10.1037//0033-2909.125.3.367. See also Amanda Eng, Andrea 't Mannetje, Dave McLean, Lis Ellison-Loschmann, Soo Cheng, and Neil Pearce, "Gender Differences in Occupational Exposure Patterns," *Occupational Environmental Medicine* 68, no. 12 (2011): 888-894, http://researchonline.lshtm.ac.uk/20521/1/workforce_survey_gender-2.pdf.

55   For a closer look at how marriage and children influence injury, see: Caroline Uggla and Ruth Mace, "Someone to Live for: Effects of Partner and Dependent Children on Preventable Death in a Population Wide Sample from Northern Ireland," *Evolution and Human Behavior* 36, no. 1 (January 2015): 1-7, https://doi.org/10.1016/j.evolhumbehav.2014.07.008 and Elizabeth L. Daugherty, Trish M. Perl, Dale M. Needham, Lewis Rubinson, Andrew Bilderback, and Cynthia S. Rand, "The Use of Personal Protective Equipment for Control of Influenza Among Critical Care Clinicians: A Survey Study," *Critical Care Medicine* 37 (2009):1210 −1216, https://pdfs.semanticscholar.org/95f2/500ab28f84e9c7e0e44e43cbce7671c8cc05.pdf.

56   Todd Grover, "Simple Ways to Improve Your Facility Lockout Practices," *EHS Today*, October 13, 2015, https://www.ehstoday.com/lockout-practices.

57   United Steelworkers, *Behavior-Based Safety/'Blame-the-Worker' Safety Program: Understanding and Confronting Management's Plan for Workplace Health and Safety* (April 2010), http://images.usw.org/conv2011/convention2011/healthsafety/Confronting%20 Blame%20the%20Worker%20Safety%20Programs%20Book%20April%202010.pdf.

58   "Gamification and Hand Safety." Superior Glove. Accessed October 23, 2019. https://www.superiorglove.com/blog/gamification-and-hand-safety.

59   *Ibid.*

60   Thomas R. Krause, *The Behavior-Based Safety Process: Managing Involvement for an Injury-Free Culture (2nd ed)* (New York: Wiley, 2000).

61   Wanda V. Myers, Terry E. McSween, Rixio E. Medina, Kristen Rost, and Alicia M. Alvero, "The Implementation and Maintenance of a Behavioral Safety Process in a Petroleum Refinery," *Journal of Organizational Behavior Management* 30, no. 4 (2010): 285-307, https://www.tandfonline.com/doi/abs/10.1080/01608061.2010.499027.

62   Some examples of evidence of success from other BBS programs include:

    1) A significant reduction in injury rates in a manufacturing plant in Mexico, compared to a control group (Jaime A. Hermann, Guillermo V. Ibarra, and B. L. Hopkins, "A Safety Program that Integrated Behavior-Based Safety and Traditional Safety Methods and Its Effects on Injury Rates of Manufacturing Workers," *Journal of Organizational Behavior Management* 30, no. 1 (2010): 6-25, https://doi.org/10.1080/01608060903472445.)

    2) An 8 percent increase in safety performance scores in 6 weeks at construction sites in Hong Kong (Rafiq M. Choudhry, "Behavior-Based Safety on Construction Sites: A Case Study." *Accident Analysis & Prevention* 70 (2014): 14-23, https://doi.org/10.1016/j.aap.2014.03.007.)

    3) The safety performance index at a large construction site in Iran increased from 66% to 92% (Morteza Oostakhan, Amirabbas Mofidi, and Amirhosain Davudian Talab, "Behavior-Based Safety Approach at a Large Construction Site in Iran," *Iranian Rehabilitation Journal* 10 (2012): 21-25, http://irj.uswr.ac.ir/files/site1/user_files_055690/admin-A-10-1-68-a42a1b9.pdf.)

63   U.S. Chemical Safety and Hazard Investigation Board, *Case Study: AL Solutions, Inc., New Cumberland, WV Metal Dust Explosion and Fire,* July 2014, https://www.csb.gov/al-solutions-fatal-dust-explosion/.

64   According to History.com, "Second officer David Blair, who held the key to the Titanic's store of binoculars in his pocket, was transferred off the ship before it left for its maiden voyage from Southampton and forgot to hand over the key to the officer who replaced him. At a later inquiry into the sinking, a lookout on the Titanic said binoculars might have helped them spot and dodge the iceberg in time. Blair kept the key as a memento of his near miss; it was auctioned off in 2007 and fetched some £90,000. See Sarah Pruitt, "Why Did the Titanic Sink?" *History,* A&E Television Networks, April 12, 2018, https://www.history.com/news/why-did-the-titanic-sink.

65   HW Heinrich, *Industrial Accident Prevention: a Scientific Approach* (4th ed.) (New York: McGraw-Hill, 1959).

66   A lost workday rate of 1.24 means that about 1.24 people out of every 100 are getting hurt so bad each day that they can't come back to work the next day. (# injuries/year x 200,000 man-hours) / (# employees x 40 hrs/wk x 50 hrs/yr) = lost workday rate

67   Douglas R. Conant, "How We Reduced Our Injury Rate by 90% at Campbell Soup Company," *Harvard Business Review*, September 5, 2018, https://hbr.org/2018/09/how-we-reduced-our-injury-rate-by-90-at-campbell-soup-company.

68   *Ibid.*

69   Charter Partners, "Paul O'Neill CEO of Alcoa - It's all about safety," YouTube video, June 12, 2015, https://www.youtube.com/watch?v=tC2ucDs_XJY.

70   James A. Klein, "Two Centuries of Process Safety at DuPont," *American Institute of Chemical Engineers Process Safety Progress* 28, (2009): 114-122, https://aiche.onlinelibrary.wiley.com/doi/pdf/10.1002/prs.10309.

71   Winston P. Ledet, "The Principles Driving Safety & Reliability: A Look at the History of DuPont," *ReliabilityWeb.com*, https://reliabilityweb.com/articles/entry/the_principles_driving_safety_reliability_a_look_at_the_history_of_dup, accessed July 11, 2019.

72   *Ibid.*

73   R. Flin and S. Yule, "Leadership for Safety: Industrial Experience," *BMJ Quality & Safety* 13 (2004):ii45-ii51, https://qualitysafety.bmj.com/content/13/suppl_2/ii45.

74   "Senior Managers View the Workplace More Positively Than Front-Line Workers," *American Psychological Association News Release*, May 12, 2015, https://www.apa.org/news/press/releases/2015/05/senior-managers.

75   Rigid Lifelines, "Emphasizing Workplace Safety Increases, Not Decreases, Your Productivity," *Fall Protection Forum*, October 18, 2017, https://www.rigidlifelines.com/blog/entry/emphasizing-workplace-safety-increases-not-decreases-your-productivity. (Original research: Aberdeen Group, *Machine Safety: The Correlation Between Safety Systems and Productivity*, March 2012, https://www.industry.siemens.nl/topics/nl/nl/safety-integrated/machineveiligheid/Documents/White_Paper_Machine_Safety_and_Productivity_2012_Aberdeen_Group.pdf.)

76   Workers' Compensation Board of British Columbia, *Lost Lives: Work-Related Deaths in British Columbia* (1999), https://www.worksafebc.com/en/resources/health-safety/report/lost-lives-workrelated-deaths-in-british-columbia-1998-98?lang=en&direct.

77   Michael Harris, "Neuroscience Confirms We Buy on Emotion & Justify with Logic & Yet We Sell to Mr. Rational & Ignore Mr. Intuitive," *Customer Think*, April 2, 2017, http://customerthink.com/neuroscience-confirms-we-buy-on-emotion-justify-with-logic-yet-we-sell-to-mr-rational-ignore-mr-intuitive/.

78 Michael Johannesson (Western Canadian sales manager at Superior Glove), in discussion with interviewer, January 29, 2019.

79 The Ikea Effect was first described by Michael I. Norton of Harvard Business School in 2009, followed up with three experiments showing that self-assembly impacts the evaluation of a product by its consumers. They concluded that when people build something themselves, they value the end product more than if they had someone else build it for them. See Michael I. Norton, "The IKEA Effect: When Labor Leads to Love," *Harvard Business Review*, February 2009, 30, http://www.people.hbs.edu/mnorton/norton%20ikea%20hbr.pdf.

80 Jon Jecker and David Landy, "Liking a Person as a Function of Doing Him a Favour," *Human Relations* 22, no. 4 (August 1, 1969): 371–378, doi:10.1177/001872676902200407.

81 Shana Lebowitz, "Harness the Power of the 'Ben Franklin Effect' to Get Someone to Like You," *Business Insider*, December 2, 2016, https://www.businessinsider.com/ben-franklin-effect-2016-12.

82 For more on the return on injury prevention dollars, see Kyle W. Morrison, "The ROI of Safety," *Safety and Health Magazine*, May 23, 2014, https://www.safetyandhealthmagazine.com/articles/10414-the-roi-of-safety.

83 Timothy Ludwig, *Dysfunctional Practices that Kill your Safety Culture (and What to Do About Them)*, (Blowing Rock, NC: Calloway Publishing, 2018).

84 *Ibid.*

85 Richard Millington, "How Quickly Can You Create a New Social Norm?" *Feverbee*, February 18, 2016, https://www.feverbee.com/norm/.

86 Jill R. Horwitz, Brenna D. Kelly, and John E. DiNardo, "Wellness Incentives in the Workplace: Cost Savings Through Cost Shifting to Unhealthy Workers," *Health Affairs* 32, no. 3 (2013): 468-476, https://www.healthaffairs.org/doi/pdf/10.1377/hlthaff.2012.0683.

87 Mark Fleming and Ronny Lardner, "Promoting Best Practice in Behavior-Based Safety," in *Hazards XVI: Analysing the Past, Planning the Future, IChemE Symposium Series No. 148* (Warwickshire, UK, Institution of Chemical Engineers, 2001): 473-486.

88 Patrick Foster and Stuart Hoult, "The Safety Journey: Using a Safety Maturity Model for Safety Planning and Assurance in the UK Coal Mining Industry," *Minerals* 3, no. 1 (2013): 59-72, http://www.mdpi.com/2075-163X/3/1/59/htm.

89 Joanne Zaraliakos, "Strategically Reduce Hand Injuries Using the Hierarchy of Hazard Control," *Iron & Steel Technology*, 2013, 41-43, https://www.aist.org/AIST/aist/AIST/Publications/safety%20first/13_augSafety_First.pdf.

90 E.B., "What "Broken Windows" Policing Is," *The Economist*, January 27, 2015, https://www.economist.com/the-economist-explains/2015/01/27/what-broken-windows-policing-is.

91 Jorma Saari and Merja Näsänen, "The Effect of Positive Feedback on Industrial Housekeeping and Accidents: A Long-Term Study at a Shipyard," *International Journal of Industrial Ergonomics* 4, no. 3 (1989): 201-211, https://www.sciencedirect.com/science/article/abs/pii/0169814189900036.

92 Unfortunately the enforcement of safety guard violations has apparently been negligible. For some references, see: Norm Keith, "After 10 Years, Bill C-45 Yields Few Prosecutions," *Canadian Occupational Safety*, April 23, 2014, https://www.cos-mag.com/ohs-laws-regulations/columns/after-10-years-bill-c-45-yields-few-prosecutions/, also David Sarvadi and Manesh Rath, "Recent Developments in OSHA Criminal Enforcement Practices," *OSHA 30/30*, June 22, 2016, https://www.khlaw.com/Files/27151_2016%20 06%2022%20DOJ%20Criminal%20Enforcement%20Memo.pdf, and also Michelle Morra, "Gotcha! There's No Hiding from the Machine Guarding Requirement," *Manufacturing Automation*, September 1, 2008, https://www.automationmag.com/factory/699-gotcha-theres-no-hiding-from-the-machine-guarding-requirement.

93 Alex Johnson, "Bumble Bee to Pay $6 Million Over Employee Cooked in Tuna Oven," *NBC News*, August 13, 2015, https://www.nbcnews.com/news/us-news/bumble-bee-pay-6-million-over-employee-cooked-tuna-oven-n408721.

94 The specifics of the OSHA safety sign standards can be found here: https://www.osha.gov/laws-regs/regulations/standardnumber/1910/1910.145. For an excellent, illustrated guide to implementing the standards, see "New OSHA/ANSI Safety Sign Systems for Today's Workplaces: A Clarion Implementation Guide," *Clarion Safety Systems*, 2013, https://www.ishn.com/ext/resources/Resources/white-papers/Clarion_ISHN_Whitepaper.pdf.

95 Thanks to safety experts Angela Lambert and Derek Eversdyke for this note. Their company helped design new alligator signs, depicted here, for Disney World in Florida after the tragedy involving a small child and an alligator on the Disney property. Angela Lambert and Derek Eversdyke, Clarion Safety Systems, personal communication, December 5, 2018.

96 Angela Lambert and Derek Eversdyke, Clarion Safety Systems, personal communication, December 5, 2018.

97 Gary S. Sorock, David A. Lombardi, David K. Peng, Russ Hauser, Ellen A. Eisen, Robert F. Herrick, and Murray A. Mittleman, "Glove Use and the Relative Risk of Acute Hand Injury: A Case-Crossover Study," *Journal of Occupational and Environmental Hygiene*, 1, no. 3 (April 2004): 182–190, https://www.tandfonline.com/doi/abs/10.1080/15459620490424500.

98 Need an ROI calculator for glove costs? See my company's website at https://www.superiorglove.com/en/roi-calculator.

99 To be a little fairer to this PM: His company supplies parts to major automakers like Ford and GM. These automakers often demand yearly cost reductions from their suppliers, like: "We want you to reduce your prices to us by 3 percent every year, across the board." They make these demands without regard to safety considerations, and of course, it's the remote workers, off their own books, who suffer most.

100 Matthew Hallowell (professor, University of Colorado Boulder), in discussion with interviewer, July 6, 2018.

101 David A.Lombardi, Gary S. Sorock, Russ Hauser, Philip C. Nasca, Ellen A. Eisen, Robert F. Herrick, and Murray A. Mittleman, "Temporal Factors and the Prevalence of Transient Exposures at the Time of an Occupational Traumatic Hand Injury," *Journal of Occupational and Environmental Medicine* 45, no. 8 (2003): 832-840, https://journals.lww.com/joem/Abstract/2003/08000/Temporal_Factors_and_the_Prevalence_of_Transient.8.aspx.

102 Matthew Hallowell (professor, University of Colorado Boulder), in discussion with interviewer, July 6, 2018.

103 In February 2019, for example, three paint buckets shoved under a display at a museum at the Grand Canyon were found to contain radioactive soil, exposing museum visitors to dangerous levels of radiation, possibly for decades. See Dennis Wagner, "Grand Canyon Tourists Exposed for Years to Radiation in Museum Building, Safety Manager Says," *Arizona Republic*, February 18, 2019, https://www.azcentral.com/story/news/local/arizona/2019/02/18/grand-canyon-tourists-exposed-radiation-safety-manager-says/2876435002/.

104 See, for example, "Mr. D: Wood Shop Saw Safety," YouTube Video, 2016, https://www.youtube.com/watch?v=4yoq4y8oP_A.

105 Ruth Colvin Clark, "More Than Just Eye Candy: Graphics for e-Learning," *The e-Learning Developers' Journal*, August 11, 2003, http://www.clarktraining.com/content/articles/MoreThanEyeCandy_part1.pdf.

106 Heesun Wee, "Korean Culture May Offer Clues in Asiana Crash," *CNBC*, July 9, 2013, https://www.cnbc.com/id/100869966.

107 Marie-Claire Ross, "King's Cross station - A Safety Accident Case Study," *Workplace Communicator Blog*, December 8, 2013, http://www.digicast.com.au/blog/bid/100338/King-s-Cross-station-A-Safety-Accident-Case-Study.

108 Tom W. Reader & Paul O'Connor, "The Deepwater Horizon Explosion: Non-Technical Skills, Safety Culture, and System Complexity," *Journal of Risk Research* 17, No. 3, (2014): 405-424, DOI: 10.1080/13669877.2013.815652.

109 Sheila McNulty, "Faults at BP Led to One of Worst US Industrial Disasters," *Financial Times*, December 18, 2006, https://www.ft.com/content/b77c5102-8ec1-11db-a7b2-0000779e2340.

110 Indeed, in the follow-up report on the disaster, issued in 2012, investigators began calling for the use of forward-looking "process safety indicators" like timely checks on safety-critical equipment. One investigator pointed out that "…the emphasis on personal injury and lost work time data obscures the bigger picture…companies need to developer indicators that give them realistic information about their potential for catastrophic accidents. How safety is measured and managed is at the very core of accident prevention. If companies are not measuring safety performance effectively and using those data to continuously improve, they will likely be left in the dark about their safety risk." See "CSB Investigation: At the Time of 2010 Gulf Blowout, Transocean, BP, Industry Associations, and Government Offshore Regulators Had Not Effectively Learned Critical Lessons from 2005 BP Refinery Explosion in Implementing Safety Performance Indicators," *CSB News Release*, July 24, 2012, https://www.csb.gov/csb-investigation-at-the-time-of-2010-gulf-blowout-transocean-bp-industry-associations-and-government-offshore-regulators-had-not-effectively-learned-critical-lessons-from-2005-bp-refinery-explosion-in-implementing-safety-performance-indicators/.

111 The OSHA regulations on recording and reporting occupational injuries and illnesses are documented at https://www.osha.gov/enforcement/directives/cpl-02-00-135.

112 This interview is insightful as to the legacy of David Michaels: Tom Musick, "Long Run: An Interview with OSHA's David Michaels," *Safety and Health Magazine*, June 26, 2016, https://www.safetyandhealthmagazine.com/articles/14298-long-run-an-interview-with-oshas-david-michaels.

113 J. Paul Leigh, "Economic Burden of Occupational Injury and Illness in the United States," *The Milbank Quarterly*, 89, No. 4, (December 2011), p. 728, http://onlinelibrary.wiley.com/doi/10.1111/j.1468-0009.2011.00648.x/abstract.

114 Michelle Chen, "Until Last Year, No One Was Tracking Workplace Injuries," *The Nation*, March 22, 2016, https://www.thenation.com/article/until-last-year-no-one-was-tracking-workplace-injuries/.

115 Occupational Safety and Health Administration, *Using Leading Indicators to Improve Safety and Health Outcomes*, June 2019, https://www.osha.gov/leadingindicators/docs/OSHA_Leading_Indicators_Guidance-07-03-2019.pdf.

116 "Frequently Asked Questions—Lagging and Leading Indicators," Safe Work Manitoba, Accessed August 18, 2019, https://www.safemanitoba.com/safetyculture/Documents/Lagging-Leading-Indicators_FAQs.pdf.

117 "Practical Guide to Leading Indicators: Metrics, Case Studies & Strategies," National Safety Council and Campbell Institute, Last modified March 5, 2015, http://www.nsc.org/CambpellInstituteandAwardDocuments/WP-PracticalGuidetoLI.pdf.

118 Gary S. Sorock, et al., "Three Perspectives on Work-Related Injury Surveillance Systems," *American Journal of Industrial Medicine*, 32, No. 2 (1997): 116-128, doi:10.1002/(SICI)1097-0274(199708)32:2<116::AID-AJIM3>3.0.CO;2-X.

119 Cary Usrey, "Reduce Incidents with Universal Metrics for Leau.. _Industrial Safety & Hygiene News_, February 1, 2018, https://www.ishn.cu.. articles/108159-reduce-incidents-with-universal-metrics-for-leading-indicators.

120 Sorock et al., "Three Perspectives…," 1997.

121 Thomas R. Krause and Kristen J. Bell, _7 Insights Into Safety Leadership_. Safety Leadership Institute: 2015.

122 _Ibid._

123 Judy Agnew and Aubrey Daniels, "Developing High-Impact Leading Indicators for Safety," Aubrey Daniels International, Accessed August 19, 2019, https://www.aubreydaniels.com/ media-center/developing-high-impact-leading-indicators-safety.

124 Danielle Kretschmer (Workforce and Leadership Development Consultant, Transformation Systems, Inc.), in discussion with interviewer, June 28, 2018.

125 "This Coach Improved Every Tiny Thing by 1 Percent and Here's What Happened," James Clear, Accessed August 19, 2019, https://jamesclear.com/marginal-gains.

126 Charles Piper (EHS manager, Exide Technologies), in discussion with interviewer, October 12, 2018.